GROWING UP SIRTFOOD DIET

2 books in 1

Sirtfood Diet for Beginners+Cookbook

A Practical Guide with Over 220 Recipes, for Children Growing up Battling Obesity and Their Families Struggling Along with Them.

ADELE FUNG

Table of content
THE SIRTFOOD DIET FOR BEGINNERS

THE SIRTFOOD DIET COOKBOOK

THE SIRTFOOD DIET FOR BEGINNERS

The simple guide with solutions for men and women, including meal plans and recipes for losing weightfast. Discover the foods that turn on your so-called skinny genes.

Adele Fung

Introduction

Fasting-based diets have become very popular over the past few years. In fact, studies show that by fasting – that is, with moderate daily calorie restriction or by practising a more radical, but less frequent, intermittent fast – you can expect to lose about 3kg in six months and substantially reduce the risk of contracting certain diseases.

When we fast, the reduction of energy reserves activates the so-called "skinny gene", which causes several positive changes. The accumulation of fat stops and the body blocks normal growth processes and enters the "survival" mode. Fats burn faster, and the genes that repair and rejuvenate cells are activated. As a result, we lose weight and increase our resistance to diseases.

All this, however, has a price. Lower energy intake leads to hunger, irritability, exhaustion and loss of muscle mass and this is a problem, the main problem, with fasting-based diets: when they are followed correctly, they work, but they make us feel so bad that we cannot repeat them. The question, then, is the following: is it possible to obtain the same results without having to impose that drastic drop in calories and, therefore, without suffering the negative consequences?

According to the sirtfood diet, it is. In fact, there is a skinny gene that, if activated properly, allows you to lose weight and gain health altogether. The singer Adele has lost 30kg in a year thanks to this philosophy: a prog of two medical nutritionists, Aidan Goggins and Glen Matten, which is based on the introduction of some sirtfoods in our diet.

These are particularly nutrient-rich foods capable of activating the same skinny genes stimulated by fasting. These genes are called sirtuins and considered to be super regulators of metabolism to influence our ability to burn fat.

This book is your sirt diet know-it-all guide. It will guide you through fun and straightforward sirt recipes that will have you shedding fat daily.

Chapter 1: What is a sirtfood?

The sirtfood diet focuses on ingredients experts say can help you live longer and turbocharge weight loss. These foods are full of components that activate the skinny gene sirtuins, which in turn revs up your weight loss. Sirtuins are a type of protein involved in regulating essential processes such as metabolism and cellular death. The breakthrough for this diet emerged when researchers discovered the benefits of fasting that come from the activation of our sirtuins gene.

When there is a shortage of energy, your body goes under stress detected by the sirtuins. The sirtuins then activate and subsequently broadcast strong signals that change the behaviour of our cells in a way that fosters a healthier, fitter, and leaner you.

"Sirtfood" is food with a high content of sirtuin activators. The word "sirt" in "sirtfood" is an abbreviation for the enzyme group of sirtuins.

While the popular low carb diet is full of proteins and allows only a small amount of carbohydrates, the sirt diet focuses on sirtuins. These are enzymes in the body that protect the cells in the body from stress through their unique activity, namely reducing the production of free radicals. If the body absorbs enough sirtuin activators from food, it also burnsfat.

The advantage: sirtuin activators are contained in a wide variety of foods and beverages, including luxury foods, and thus enable a varied diet that is not very restrictive. The only task in this diet is to consume as many foods as possible that are rich in these sirtuinactivators.

Sirtuins strengthen the immune system, help build muscle and ensure that cell metabolism decreases – in other words, the ageing process slows down, you stay "young longer". All you need to do is switch to foods that activate many sirtuins.

Sirtuins not only make you young and healthy but also slim. The promise of the sirtuin diet: within one week, you can lose up to 3kg. If you also exercise more and burn calories, you can become even slimmer in this short period; because the more muscles you have, the more calories you burn. Sirtuin-activating foods also inhibit ravenous appetite attacks.

The best-known woman that the sirt diet has helped is none other than singer Adele.

The sirtfood diet depends on the possibility that specific nourishments initiate sirtuins in your body, which are specific proteins conjectured to receive different rewards, from shielding cells in your body from aggravation to turning around maturing. Nourishments permitted on a diet incorporate green tea, dull chocolate, apples, natural citrus products, parsley, turmeric, kale, blueberries, tricks and red wine.

On the authority sirtfood diet site, defenders clarify that the diet has two "simple" stages. Stage one is seven days with every day comprising of three sirtfood green juices and one dinner loaded up with sirtfoods – an aggregate of 1,000 calories. Yet, don't be disheartened: you may be somewhat less starving on days four through seven when you're permitted to build your admission to 1,500 calories with two green juices and two dinners. Phew!

Stage two isn't considerably more encouraging. This stage goes on for about fourteen days, in which you are allowed to have three "adjusted" sirtfood-rich dinners every day notwithstanding your one unique green juice. The objective during this time is to advance further weight loss. While the advantages of sirtuins appear to be encouraging, the sirtfood diet is showcased up until now another approach to "shed seven pounds in seven days!" and you know at this point extreme diets simply don't work that way.

Here are three motivations to take a pass on the sirtfood diet:

1. The sirtfood diet estimates achievement just as far as weight loss.

Weight is a determinant of wellbeing, yet it's not alone. To gauge somebody's wellbeing accomplishment on whether they lose 'x' pounds in 'x' measure of time overlooks the various advantages of nourishment. Nourishment is brimming with vitality, which enables you to do things like showering, practising and relaxing. It additionally has supplements that can advance a few substantial capacities and is often a cheerful encounter established in custom. For by and large wellbeing, there's a great deal more to concentrate on than basically appearance, and estimating achievement just as far as weight loss is incomprehensive.

2. It's prohibitive, which can harm your association with nourishment.

This diet stresses an admission of 1,000 to 1,500 calories for every day, which is a lot of lower than a great many people need. When we seriously limit our nourishment admission, our intuitive response is to indulge. Your body is savvy, and it thinks about this absence of sustenance as an assault. Therefore, we will in general overcompensate, which is the reason we as a whole can identify with being "hangry" and thus overindulging when we're at last allowed to eat. Rehearsing careful and intuitive eating is a more practical course than confining nourishment.

3. The sirtfood diet isn't science-based.

While there is some questionable research about the advantages of sirtuins, there's practically zero research about the specific sirtfood diet. Moreover, we, as of now, have a few rules set up that have been thoroughly looked into and tried for quite a long time. If you're lost on what "sound nourishment" is, this is a superior spot to begin.

It's fine if you need to join a couple sirtfoods into an eating plan. Nourishments like green tea, organic product, dim chocolate and kale all include a spot inside a smart dieting design! Be that as it may, holding fast to a prog with such exacting pass-or-bomb prerequisites is unreasonable and could be hurtful to your association with nourishment. By fusing an eating plan that is loaded with assortment and eating carefully, you'll have the option to set up a long haul, manageable association with nourishment. Cheers to that!

What to know before start sirtfood diet

"Sirtfood" seems like something created by outsiders, brought to earth for human utilisation with expectations of picking up mind control and global control. In fact, sirtfoods are essentially nourishments high in sirtuins. Uh, come again? Sirtuins are a sort of protein that reviews on natural product flies, and mice have indicated control digestion, increment bulk and consume fat.

As indicated by the book, this arrangement can assist you with consuming fat and lift your vitality, preparing your body for long haul weight-loss achievement and a more drawn out more beneficial ailment free life and all that while drinking red wine. Sounds like practically the ideal diet, isn't that so? All things considered, before you consume your reserve funds loading up on sirtuins-filled fixings, read the upsides and downsides.

The underlying power of sirtfoods

Sirtfoods are simply foods that activate the sirtuin genes. These foods are unique for this function because they contain a natural plant chemical known as polyphenols. This chemical 'speaks' to the sirtuin genes and switches them on. Polyphenols are dietary antioxidants that help decrease the development of fat cells and reduce fatty tissue – they mimic the effects of fasting or exercising.

Because they are stationary, plants have developed a sophisticated stress response system. They produce polyphenols to help them adapt to harsh environments. By consuming these plants, we benefit from the effects that activate our innate stress response pathways.

All plants have these response systems, but only certain plants produce a significant amount of the sirtuin-activating polyphenol. Discovery of these foods means you can lose weight through eating sirtfoods.

What is so great about sirtuins?

There are seven types of sirtuins named from *sirt1* to *sirt7*. Although our understanding of the exact functions of all the sirtuins is minimal, studies show that activating them can have the following benefits:

- *Switching on fat burning and protection from weight gain:* sirtuins do this by increasing the functionality of the mitochondrion (which is involved in the production of energy) and sparking a change in your metabolism to break down more fatcells.
- The activated sirts increase the amount of a neurotransmitter known as norepinephrine used as a signal to fat cells. These transmitters tell the fat cells to breakdown fat and convert into energy.
- *Improving memory* by protecting neurons from damage. Sirtuins also boost learning skills and memory through the enhancement of synaptic plasticity. Synaptic plasticity refers to the ability of synapses to weaken or strengthen with time due to decrease or increase in their activity. This is important because memories are represented by different interconnect network of synapses in the brain and synaptic plasticity is an important neurochemical foundation of memory and learning.
- *Slowing down the ageing process:* sirtuins act as cell guarding enzymes. Thus, they protect the cells and slow down their ageing process.
- *Repairing cells:* the sirtuins repair cells damaged by re-activating cellfunctionality.
- *Protection against diabetes:* this happens through prevention against insulin resistance. Sirtuins do this by controlling blood sugar levels because this diet calls for moderate consumption of carbohydrates. These foods cause increases in blood sugar levels; hence the need to release insulin and as the blood sugar levels increase greatly there is need to produce more insulin. Over time, cells become resistant to insulin; hence, the need to produce more insulin and this leads to insulinresistance.
- *Fighting cancers:* the chemicals working as sirtuin activators affect the function of sirtuin in different cells, *i.e.* By switching it on when in normal cells and shutting it down in cancerous cells. This encourages the death of cancerous cells.
- *Fighting inflammation:* sirtuins have a powerful antioxidant effect that has the power to reduce oxidative stress. This has positive effects on heart health and cardiovascular protection.

Food list

Sirtfoods list in addition to red wine and chocolate allowed in this diet, here are other foods included:

Apples	Blueberries
Capers	Celery
Chilli	Citrus fruits
Coffee	Dates
Fruits and	Kale
Lovage	Medjool
Onions	Parsley
Passion fruit	Red chicory
Rocket	Soy
Strawberries	Tofu
Turmeric	Vegetables
Walnuts	

Red wine in this diet steals the limelight because it is rich in sirtuins and because it is most people's favourite type of drink.

chocolate contains sirtuin-activating antioxidant resveratrol. You should opt for dark chocolate rather than milk chocolate, however, for the greatest benefit, opt for baking chocolate or cocoa powder, which contain more resveratrol than all ready to eat chocolates.

Olive oil has a sufficient amount of the sirt activator oleuropein. To get the best out of olive oil, use extra virgin olive oil (EVOO). The benefits of the oil start at 2 tbsp a day.

Green tea contains a phytochemical known as epigallocatechin-3-gallate (egcg) known to activate and control sirtuins directly to anti-cancer action. Preferably, drink matcha green ta because it contains three times more egcg than other brands of green tea.

Now that you know what the sirtfood diet is, the function of sirtuins, how sirtuins help the body lose weight, as well as the foods you should reach for, the rest of the guide shall revolve around giving you easy and delicious sirtfood diet recipes.

The taste does not tell us which food contains sirtuin – it is found in bitter fruits and vegetables as well as in sweets. For this reason, we have created a small overview of foods that contain sirtuin.

Of course, you do not have to limit yourself to the following list of foods. The aim is to include the delicacies containing sirtuin in the menu as often as possible. For luxury goods such as coffee, chocolate or red wine, the following applies: always enjoy with care and do not eat or drink too much.

20 most important sirtfoods:

Arugula	Buckwheat
Capers	Celery
Chillies (birds eye chilli)	Cocoa (pure or in 85% chocolate)
Coffee	Dates (Medjoul)
Green tea	Kale
Lovage	Olive oil
Onions (red)	Parsley
Radicchio	Red wine
Soya	Strawberries
Turmeric	Walnuts

The following 40 other sirtuin-activating foods are also recommended in the sirtfood diet. These are not quite as strongly activating as those from the top 20 list but are still highly recommended.

Fruits

apples · blackberries · cranberries · goji berries · raspberries · currants (black) · kumquats · plums · grapes (red)

Vegetables and legumes

artichokes · broccoli · watercress · chicory (light) · broad beans · white beans · green beans · last salad · bok choy · shallots · asparagus · onions (white)

Beverages

black tea · white tea

Cereals

popcorn · quinoa · wholemeal flour

Herbs and spices

chilli · dill · ginger · mint · oregano · legend · chives · thyme

Nuts and seeds

chia seeds · peanuts · chestnuts · pecan nuts · pistachios · sunflower seeds

How can it work?

At its centre, the way to getting in shape is really basic: create a calorie shortage either by expanding your calorie consume exercises or diminishing your caloric admission. Be that as it may, imagine a scenario where you could avoid the dieting and rather actuate a "thin quality" without the requirement for extraordinary calorie limitation. This is the reason for the sirtfood diet, composed by nourishment specialists Aidan Goggins and Glen Matten. The best approach to do it, they contend, is sirtfoods.

Sirtfoods are wealthy in supplements that enact a purported "thin quality" called sirtuin. As indicated by Goggins and Matten, the "thin quality" is enacted when a lack of vitality is made after you confine calories. Sirtuins got intriguing to the sustenance world in 2003 when scientists found that resveratrol, a compound found in red wine, had a similar impact on life length as calorie limitation yet it was accomplished without decreasing admission. (Discover the conclusive truth about wine and its medical advantages.)

In the 2015 pilot study (led by Goggins and Matten) testing the adequacy of sirtuins, the 39 members lost a normal of seven pounds in seven days. Those outcomes sound amazing, yet it's imperative to understand this is a small example size concentrated over a brief timeframe. Weight-loss specialists additionally have their questions about the elevated guarantees. "The cases made are theoretical and extrapolate from considers which were generally centred around straightforward creatures (like yeast) at the cell level. What occurs at the cell level doesn't mean what occurs in the human body at the large scale level," says Adrienne Youdim, m.d., the chief of the Centre for Weight Loss and Nutrition in Beverly Hills, CA. (Here, look at the best and most exceedingly awful diets to follow this year.)

The diet is executed in two stages. Stage one endures three days and limits calories to 1,000 every day, comprising of three green juices and one sirtfood-endorsed supper. Stage two keeps going four days and raises the everyday designation to 1,500 calories for each day with two green juices and two dinners.

After these stages, there is an upkeep plan that isn't centred around calories yet rather on reasonable bits, well-adjusted suppers, and topping off on principally sirtfoods. The 14-day upkeep plan highlights three dinners, one green juice, and a couple sirtfood chomp snacks. Adherents are additionally urged to finish 30 minutes of movement five days per week-per government proposals; however, it isn't the fundamental focal point of the arrangement.

What are the advantages?

You will get thinner if you follow this diet intently. "Regardless of whether you're eating 1,000 calories of tacos, 1,000 calories of kale, or 1,000 calories of snickerdoodles, you will get in shape at 1,000 calories!" says dr. Youdim. In any case, she additionally calls attention to that you can have accomplishment with an increasingly sensible calorie limitation. "The run of the mill every day caloric admission of somebody not on a diet is 2,000 to 2,200, so lessening to 1,500 is as yet limiting and would be a powerful weight-loss procedure for most," she says.

Sirtfood Allergy labels:

Sf – soy-free   Gf – gluten-free

Df – dairy-free   Ef – egg-free

V – vegan   Nf – nut-free

Are there any safeguards?

"This arrangement is severe with little squirm room or substitutions, and weight loss must be kept up if the low caloric admission is additionally kept up, making it difficult to cling to the long haul. That implies any weight you lost in the initial seven days is probably going to be recovered after you finish," says dr. Youdin. Her primary concern is "restricting protein consumption with juices will bring about a loss of bulk. Losing muscle is synonymous with dropping your metabolic rate or 'digestion,' making weight upkeep progressively difficult," she says.

Chapter 2: How the sirtfood diet works

Singer Adele has confirmed that she has lost 30kg in just one year. The secret? It's all thanks to the sirtfood diet. The singer herself revealed it through international media, such as the daily mail and the new york post.

The sirtfood diet is not the classic fasting diet: Adele is the living proof of this, given the splendid shape in which was at her appointments with her fans. It is, in fact, a diet that leaves room for both cheese and red wine as well as chocolate, in the right proportions, and of course under the supervision of a specialist doctor, who knows how to evaluate your health and recommend the most suitable diet to lose weight safely.

Many were the media that underlined the substantial weight loss of the singer Adele who admitted, how the decision to lose weight did not depend on the acceptance of herself as much as the difficulty of using her voice to the fullest.

Adele praised the sirtfood diet, which made her lose 30kg without much effort (although in reality, she admitted via Instag that she had never struggled as much in physical activity as when preparing for her tour). She also said that the beauty of sirt foods is that many of them are already on our table every day. They are accessible and can be easily integrated into our diet.

Although being thinner was not her priority (the singer has always had an excellent relationship with her body), she wanted to review her eating habits to get back in shape, but also (or better above all) to feel good about herself.

Furthermore, the sirtfood diet had come back on the news because it was Pippa Middleton's choice to get back into shape quickly before her wedding with the millionaire James Matthews that was celebrated on May 20, 2017.

Pippa Middleton would have tested the concrete benefits of this hunger-free regime by eating the ingredients of the sirtfood diet prepared by nutritionists Aidan Goggins and Glen Matten with gusto. Nothing to do with the Dukan, diet followed by sister Kate before marrying Prince William, one of the many fasting diets that currently exist.

Introduction

The sirtfood diet is a diet named after a molecule in some plant-based foods, called sirtuin activators. Sirtuin activators are a type of protein that helps insulate cells from the effect of ageing, inflammation and several nasty metabolic processes.

Owing to this, sirtuin activators have been associated with longevity, with people who intake high amounts of sirtuin over long periods demonstrably living longer than their peers. There are also numerous other benefits, such as increases in muscle mass and making it easier to burn. The sirtfood diet revolves around, ensuring you keep your sirtuin intake high, promoting weight loss and overall bodily health.

The interesting part of the sirtfood diet is its shift in focus. This isn't a fad diet to lose weight – rather the emphasis is just eating in a healthy and balanced way, with weight loss naturally occurring once your body has been cleansed of your poor eating habits.

There are many foods which contain sirtuin activators, most notably both chocolate and red wine. Of course, the sirtuin diet doesn't claim to be a miracle diet where you can binge on chocolate and wine, if only hey!. You will still need to balance your intake of calories and ensure you receive an even spread of essential food groups too.

The core of the diet consists of healthy sirtuin activator foods, which includes apples, citrus fruits, blueberries, green tea, soy, strawberries, turmeric, olive oil, red onion and kale. There are also a couple of surprises, such as coffee, which is usually reprimanded in most contemporary diets.

However, the problem with fasting diets, as the name implies, is that you have to fast. Fasting feels awful, especially when we are surrounded by other people having regular eating habits. It also puts some social spotlight on your own diet – explaining to your co-workers or your extended family why you are not eating on certain days is bound to generate incredulity and challenges to your diet regime.

Furthermore, even though fasting has numerous associated benefits, there are some downsides too. Fasting is associated with muscle loss, as the body doesn't discriminate between muscle mass and fat tissue when choosing cells to burn for energy.

Fasting also risks malnutrition, simply by not eating enough foods to get essential nutrients. This risk can be somewhat alleviated by taking vitamin supplements and eating nutrient-rich foods, but fasting can also slow and halt the digestive system altogether – preventing the absorption of supplements. These supplements also need dietary fat to be dissolved, which you might also lack if you were to implement a strict fasting.

On top of this, fasting isn't appropriate for a huge range of people. Obviously, you don't want children to fast and potentially inhibit their growth. Likewise, the elderly, the ill and the pregnant are all just too vulnerable to the risks of fasting.

Additionally, there are several psychological detriments to fasting, despite commonly being associated with spiritual revelations. Fasting makes you irritable and causes you to feel slightly on edge – your body is telling you constantly that you need to forage for food, enacting physical processes that affect your mood and emotions.

This is why the authors of the sirtfood diet sought a replacement for fasting diets. Fasting is beneficial for our body, but it just isn't practical for society at large. This is where sirtuin activators and sirtfoods come to the rescue.

Sirtuins were first discovered in 1984 in yeast molecules. Of course, once it became apparent that sirtuin activators affected a variety of factors, such as lifespan and metabolic activity, interest in these proteins blossomed.

Sirtuin activators boost your mitochondria's activity, the part of the biological cell which is responsible for the production of energy. This, in turn, mirrors the energy-boosting effects, which also occur due to exercise and fasting. The sirtfood diet is thought to start a process called adipogenesis, which prevents fat cells from duplicating – which should interest any potential dieter.

The interesting part is that the sirtuin activators influence your genetics. The notion of the 'genetic' lottery is embedded in the public consciousness, but genes are more changeable then you might think. You won't be able to change your eye colour or your height, but you can activate or deactivate specific genes based on environmental factors. This is called epigenetics, and it is a fascinating field of study.

Sirtuin activators cause the sir genes to activate, the before-mentioned 'skinny genes', which in turn increases the release of sirts. Sirts or silent information regulators also help regulate the circadian rhythm, which is your natural body clock and influences sleep patterns.

Sleep is important for many vital biological processes, including those that help regulate blood sugar (which is also important for losing weight). If you find yourself constantly stuck in a state of lag and brain fog, this may be caused by your circadian rhythm being out of sync, which is another way the sirtfood diet can help your body.

Additionally, sirts help contain free radicals. Free radicals are not as awesome as the sound – they are a.w.o.l particles in your body that damage your DNA and speed up the ageing process.

To summarise, the sirtfood diet contains foods which are high in sirtuin activators. Sirtuin activators activate your sir genes or 'skinny genes' which enact beneficial metabolic processes. These processes, which involve molecules, called sirts, causes your body to burn fat, repair bodily cells and combat free radicals.

So, sirtfoods have been hailed as the next dietary wonder – but where is the cold, hard evidence? Well, the evidence for the sirtfood diet comes from multiple sources. To start with, Aidan Goggins and Glen Matten, the originators of the sirtfood diet, performed their own trial at a privately owned fitness centre to test sirtfoods themselves.

At a fitness centre called kx, in Chelsea, London, the two authors of the sirtfood diet made a selection of their clientèle eat a carefully monitored constructed sirtfood diet. What is particularly interesting about the study is that weight wasn't the only variable measured – the researchers also measured body composition and metabolic activity – they were searching for the holistic effect of the diet.

97.5% of people managed to stick to the first-three day fasting period, involving only 1,000 calories. Generally speaking, this is a much higher rate of success than typical fasting diets, where many people have their willpower shattered in just the first few days.

Out of the 40 participants, 39 completed the study. In terms of overall fitness and weight, the individuals in the study were well distributed – 2 were officially obese, 15 fell into the overweight category while 22 had a regular body mass index. There were also 21 women and 18 men – a diet for both the genders! However, with that being said, being members of a fitness centre, the individuals in the study were more likely to exercise more than the standard population – a potential confounding factor.

Participants lost over 7lbs on average in the first week. Every participant experienced an improvement in body composition, even if their gains were not as dramatic as their peers.

There were also numerous reported psychological benefits, although these were not formally quantified. These improvements include an overall sense of feeling and looking better. As a side note, it was also claimed the 40 participants rarely felt hungry, even despite the calorie deficits imposed by the diet.

The most startling result from the sirtfood diet is that muscle mass after the 1-week diet period was either the same as before, or showed slight improvements. Dieting law typically states that when losing fat, muscle is also lost, usually around 20-30% of the total weight loss, you should lose 2-3 lbs of muscle for every 10 lbs lost.

Of course, retaining muscle isn't just better from an overall fitness perspective, but also from an aesthetic view. A common fear, especially in men, is that if they lose weight is that they will look skinny, scrawny and unhealthy. Yet by the retaining the muscle you will gain that toned, slither look that is so fashionable in models.

Another important reason why retaining muscle mass is your resting energy expenditure. Your muscles require energy, even when you are not using them intensely. Owing to this, people who keep skeletal muscle burn more calories than people who don't, even if both people are sedentary. Basically, being muscular allows you to eat more calories and get away with it!

Muscle mass has also been associated with a general decrease in degenerative diseases as you age (such as diabetes and osteoporosis) as well as lower rates of mental health problems (such as depression and excessive anger).

Overall, the clinical trial performed at the kx fitness centre not only supported the notion that the sirtfood diet can aid weight loss and promote holistic body health, but it also leads to the surprising finding that sirtfoods can retain muscle mass.

This is the beauty of the sirtfood diet – it isn't trying to make your eating habits artificial and awkward. It is simply copying the healthiest practices that already exist around the world.

Skeletal muscle is all the muscles you voluntarily control, such as the muscles in your limbs, back, shoulders, and so on. There are two other types: cardiac muscle is what the heart is formed of, while the smooth muscle is your involuntary muscles – which includes muscles around your blood vessels, face and various parts of organs and other tissues.

Skeletal muscle is separated into two different groups, the blandly named type-1 and type-2. Type 1 muscle is effective at continued, sustained activity whereas type-2 muscle is effective at short, intense periods of activity. So, for example, you would predominantly use type-1 muscles for jogging, but type-2 muscles for sprinting.

Sirt-1 protects the type-1 muscles, but not the type-2 muscle, which is still broken down for energy. Therefore, holistic muscle mass drops when fasting, even though type-1 skeletal muscle mass increases.

Sirt-1 also influences how the muscles work. Sirt-1 is produced by the muscle cells, but the ability to produce sirt-1 decreases as the muscle ages. As a result, muscle is harder to build as you age and doesn't grow as fast in response to exercise. A lack of sirt-1 also causes the muscles to become tired quicker and gradually decline over time.

When you start to consider these effects of sirt-1, you can start to form a picture of why fasting helps keep the body supple. Fasting releases sirt-1, which in turn helps skeletal muscle grow and stay in good shape. sirt-1 is also released by consuming sirtuin activators, giving the sirtfood diet its muscle retaining power.

How much sirtfood do you need to eat?

Of course, the sirtfood diet is more than just pumping a bunch of the best sirtfoods into your eating habits. It is a holistic diet with food organised into different meals, each designed to give you the highest sirtuin kick. On top of this, the sirtfood diet isn't exotic.

The main ingredients of the sirtfood diet are common, and you probably use them already, on occasion. The trick is just making sure you are getting enough – the average American only receives 13Mg of sirtuins a day – which is five times lower than their Japanese counterparts.

So if sirtuins are so fantastic, why don't we take them as a supplement or pill? The truth is although a pharmaceutical application of sirtuins may be possible in the future, our current understanding of food science and biology is still too limited for this to be effective today.

Understanding how sirtuins are processed and absorbed, which likely depends on other nutrients in food, is crucial to making sirtuins work. At the moment, it is simply easier and more successful to consume sirtuins the natural way, receiving all the extra stuff you need in the sirtfoods themselves.

For example, resveratrol, the sirtuin activator, which is present in certain types of red wine, is known to be absorbed poorly when taken, are a pure substance. When ingested in red-wine, it is in fact absorbed six times better. Simply put, food is complicated and we only understand a few pieces of the puzzle.

Another reason why sirtuins are not taken as a pill or supplement is the fact there are so many of them, all with slightly different effects. Add this to the before-mentioned complexity, and it's better to consume foods where you know you get a natural mix.

Fortunately, this draconian restriction only lasts three days, in which you progress to a four-day stage where you are allotted another 500 calories, and you can replace one of your juices with another sirtfood meal.

Finally, after four more days you progress to phase-2, where you are allowed three full sirtfood meals and one meal juice for another two-weeks. In this period, your focus in on keeping your intake of sirtfoods high and maintaining your weight loss.

You do not need to eat a calorie deficit in phase 2, but nor should you be eating more calories than you need. The sirtfood diet claims that you can maintain weight loss during this period, even without the calorie deficit due to the changes in our body.

After the 14-day maintenance period, you have the freedom to choose your own eating habits. The sirtfood diet isn't a diet for life; rather, it is a temporary change to your eating habits intended to change how your body is processing food.

Therefore whenever you need a fat-burning boost, you can re-implement the three-stage sirtfood dieting process to speed up your weight loss and cleanse your body. Of course, over a longer period, ideally, you should gradually implement more and more sirtfoods into your lifestyle.

You should also make an effort to make sirtfood recipes practical for your family. Batch cooking and freezing will help with the constant demand to cook. Likewise, several recipes are remarkably quick and low-effort and can be used as quick solutions to hungrymouths.

The sirtfood diet was an achievement nourishment system a couple of years and was the dear eating routine with the broadsheet press at the time. If you missed it, the features are that it incorporates red wine, chocolate, and espresso. Far less promoted and eye-catching, (yet similarly uplifting news as we would like to think) is the way that the response to the inquiry, 'would you be able to eat meat on the sirt nourishment diet?', is a resonating, yes.

The eating routine arrangement not just incorporates a decent sound part of the meat; it proceeds to recommend that protein is a basic consideration in a sirtfood-based eating routine to receive the greatest reward.

We're not supporting this as some meat overwhelming eating routine (we despite everything recollect the awful breath from Atkins), it's in reality very veggie-lover cordial and provides food for practically everybody, which is the thing that makes it so reasonable an alternative to us.

So what is the sirtfood diet? Nutritionists created it Aidan Goggins and Glen Matten, following a pilot learn at the elite xk gym, (Daniel Craig, Madonna and an entire host of different celebs are supposedly individuals) where they are the two experts in Sloane Square, London. Members in the preliminary lost 7lbs in the initial seven days, in what the creators call the hyper-achievement to organise. The science behind sirtfoods drops out of an investigation in 2003 which found that a compound found in red wine, expanded the life expectancy of yeast. At last, this prompted the investigations which clarify the medical advantages of red wine, and how (whenever drank reasonably) individuals who drink red wine put on less weight.

A significant part of the science behind the sirtfood diet is like that of 'fasting-diets' which have been well known for as far back as barely any years, whereby our bodies initiate qualities and our fat stockpiling is turned off; our bodies change to endurance mode, thus weight reduction. The negatives to fasting-eats fewer carbs are the unavoidable craving that results, alongside a decrease in vitality, bad-tempered conduct (when you're "hangry"), weariness and muscle misfortune. The sirtfood diet professes to counter those negatives, as it's anything but a quick, so hunger isn't an issue, making it ideal for individuals who need to lead a functioning solid way of life.

Sirtfoods are a (generally newfound) gathering of nourishments that are incredible in actuating the 'sirtuin' qualities in our body, which are the qualities enacted in fasting eats fewer carbs. Critically for us carnivores, the book proceeds to recommend in the section entitled 'sirtfoods forever' that protein is basic to keep up digestion and decrease the loss of muscle when counting calories. Leucine is an amino corrosive found in protein, which praises and upgrades the activities of sirtfoods. This implies the most ideal approach to eat sirtfoods is by consolidating them with a chicken bosom, steak or another wellspring of leucine, for example, fish or eggs.

Generally, we can thoroughly observe the advantage and intrigue of the sirtfood diet. Like practically any eating regimen plan, it tends to be a faff getting every one of the fixings, and the 'sirtfood green juice', which shapes a centrepiece of the initial 14 days of the arrangement, is a torment to make and is costly, yet it shows improvement over you'd anticipate. We just trialled a couple of days of the arrangement and keeping in mind that there was perceptible weight reduction, the genuine advantage of the book is the reasonable Directions ology of bringing sirtfoods into your regular dinner arranging.

Chapter 3: How to follow the sirt food diet

Phase 1 of the diet is the one that produces the greatest results. Over the course of seven days, you will follow simple directions to lose 3.5kg. Following, you will find a step-by-step guide, complete with menus and recipes.

During the first three days, the intake of calories will have to be limited to 1,000 per day at most. You can have three green juices and a solid meal, all based on sirt foods. From day 4 to 7, the daily calories will become fifteen hundred. Every day you will eat two green juices and two solid sirt meals. By the end of the seven days, you should have lost, on average, 3.5kg.

Despite the reduction in calories, the participants do not feel hungry, and the calorie limit is an indication rather than a goal. Even in the most intensive phase, calorie restriction is not as drastic as in many other regimes. Sirt foods have a naturally satiating effect so that many of you will feel pleasantly full and satisfied.

Phase 2 is the maintenance phase and lasts 14 days: during this period, although the main objective is not the reduction of calories, you will consolidate weight loss and continue to lose weight. The secret to succeeding at this stage lies in continuing to eat sirt foods in abundance; following the prog that we will provide you with relative recipes will facilitate you. During those two weeks, you will consume three balanced and rich sirt foods per day and a green sirt juice.

Phase 1

Monday: 3 green juices | breakfast: water + tea or espresso + a cup of green juice; | lunch: green juice | snack: a square of dark chocolate | dinner: sirt meal | after dinner: a square of dark chocolate.

Drink the juices at three distinct times of the day (for example, in the morning as soon as you wake up, mid-morning and mid-afternoon) and choose the normal or vegan dish: pan-fried oriental prawns with buckwheat spaghetti or miso and tofu with sesame glaze and sautéed vegetables (vegan dish).

Tuesday: 3 green juices | breakfast: water + tea or espresso + a cup of green juice | lunch: 2 green juices | before dinner snack: a square of dark chocolate | dinner: sirt meal | after dinner: a square of dark chocolate.

Welcome to day 2 of the sirtfood diet. The formula is identical to that of the first day, and the only thing that changes is the solid meal. Today you will also have dark chocolate, and the same goes for tomorrow. This food is so wonderful that we don't need an excuse to eat it.

To earn the title of a "sirt food", chocolate must be at least 85% cocoa, and even among the various types of chocolate with this percentage, not all of them are the same. Often this product is treated with an alkalising agent (this is the so-called "dutch process") to reduce its acidity and give it a darker colour. Unfortunately, this process greatly reduces the flavonoids activating sirtuins, compromising their health benefits. Lindt excellence 85% chocolate, is not subjected to the dutch process and is therefore often recommended.

On day 2, capers are also included in the menu. Despite what many may think, they are not fruits, but buds that grow in Mediterranean countries and are picked by hand. They are fantastic sirt foods because they are very rich in the nutrients kaempferol and quercetin. From the point of view of flavour, they are tiny concentrates of taste. If you've never used them, don't feel intimidated. You will see, they will taste amazingly if combined with the right ingredients, and they will give an unmistakable and inimitable aroma to your dishes.

On the second day, you will intake 3 green sirt juices and 1 solid meal (normal or vegan).

Drink the juices at three distinct times of the day (for example, when you wake up in the morning, mid-morning and mid-afternoon) and choose either the normal or the vegan dish: turkey escalope with capers, parsley, and sage on spiced cauliflower couscous or curly kale and red onion dahl with buckwheat (vegan dish).

Wednesday: 3 green juices | breakfast: water + tea or espresso + a cup of green juice | lunch: 2 green juices | before dinner snack: a square of dark chocolate | dinner: sirt meal | after dinner: a square of dark chocolate.

You are now on the third day, and even if the format is once again identical to that of days 1 and 2, so the time has come to flavour everything with a fundamental ingredient. For thousands of years, chilli has been a fundamental element of the gastronomic experiences of the whole world.

If you are not a big expert of chilli, we recommend the bird's eye (sometimes called Thai chilli) because it is the best for sirtuins.

This is the last day you will consume three green juices a day; tomorrow, you will switch to two. We, therefore, take this opportunity to browse other drinks that you can have during the diet. We all know that green tea is good for health, and water is naturally very good, but what about coffee? More than half of people drink at least one coffee a day, but always with a trace of guilt because some say that it is a vice and an unhealthy habit. This is untrue; studies show that coffee is a real treasure trove of beneficial plant substances. That's why coffee drinkers run the least risk of getting diabetes, certain forms of cancer, and neurodegenerative diseases. Furthermore, not only is coffee, not a toxin, it protects the liver and makes it even healthier!

On the third day, you will intake 3 green sirt juices and 1 solid meal (normal or vegan, see below).

Drink the juices at three distinct times of the day (for example, in the morning as soon as you wake up, mid-morning and mid-afternoon) and choose the normal or vegan dish: aromatic chicken breast with kale, red onion, tomato sauce, and chilli or baked tofu with harissa on spiced cauliflower couscous (vegan dish).

Thursday: 3 green juices | breakfast: water + tea or espresso + a cup of green juice | lunch: sirt food | snack: 1 green juice before dinner | dinner: sirt food

The fourth day of the sirtfood diet has arrived, and you are halfway through your journey to a leaner and healthier body. The big change from the previous three days is that you will only drink two juices instead of three and that you will have two solid meals instead of one. This means that on the fourth day and the upcoming ones, you will have two green juices and two solid meals, all delicious and rich in sirt foods. The inclusion of Medjool dates in a list of foods that promote weight loss and good health may seem surprising. Especially when you think they contain 66% sugar.

Sugar has no stimulating properties towards sirtuins. On the contrary, it has well-known links with obesity, heart disease, and diabetes; in short, just at the antipodes of the objectives, we aim to. But industrially refined and processed sugar is very different from the sugar present in a food that also contains sirtuin-activating polyphenols: the Medjool dates. Unlike regular sugar, these dates, consumed in moderation, do not increase the level of glucose in the blood.

Today we will also integrate chicory into meals. Like with onion, red chicory is better in this case too, but endive, its close relative, is also a sirt food. If you are looking for ideas on the use of these salads, combine them with other varieties and season them with olive oil: they will give a pungent flavour to milder leaves.

On the fourth day, you will intake: 2 green sirt juices, 2 solid meals (normal or vegan) drink the juices at different times of the day (for example the first in the morning as soon as you wake up or in the middle of the morning, the second in the middle of the afternoon) and choose the normal or vegan dishes: muesli sirt, pan-fried salmon fillet with caramelised chicory, rocket salad, and celery leaves or muesli sirt and Tuscan stewed beans (vegan dish).

Friday: 2 green juices | breakfast: water + tea or espresso + a cup of green juice | lunch: sirt food | snack: a green juice before dinner | dinner: sirt food

You have reached the fifth day, and the time has come to add fruits. Due to its high sugar content, fruits have been the subject of bad publicity. This does not apply to berries. Strawberries have a very low sugar content: one tsp per 100 gs. They also have an excellent effect on how the body processes simple sugars.

Scientists have found that if we add strawberries to simple sugars, this causes a reduction in insulin demand, and therefore transforms food into a machine that releases energy for a long time. Strawberries are, therefore, a perfect element in diets that will help you lose weight and get back in shape. They are also delicious and extremely versatile, as you will discover in the sirt version of the fresh and light middle eastern tabbouleh.

Miso, made from fermented soy, is a traditional Japanese dish. Miso contains a strong umami taste, a real explosion for the taste buds. In our modern society, we know better monosodium glutamate, artificially created to reproduce the same flavour. Needless to say, it is far preferable to derive that magical umami flavour from traditional and natural food, full of beneficial substances. It is found in the form of a paste in all good supermarkets and healthy food stores and should be present in every kitchen to give a touch of taste to many different dishes.

Since umami flavours enhance each other, miso is perfectly associated with other tasty/umami foods, especially when it comes to cooked proteins, as you will discover today in the delicious, fast and easy dishes you will eat.

On the fifth day, you will intake 2 green sirt juices and 2 solid meals (normal or vegan).

Drink the juices at different times of the day (for example the first in the morning as soon as you wake up or in the middle of the morning, the second in the middle of the afternoon) and choose the normal or vegan dishes.

Saturday: 2 green juices | breakfast: water + tea or espresso + a cup of green juice | lunch: sirt food | snack: a green juice before dinner | dinner: sirt food

There are no sirt foods better than olive oil and red wine. Virgin olive oil is obtained from the fruit only by mechanical means, in conditions that do not deteriorate it, so that you can be sure of its quality and polyphenol content. "extra virgin" oil is that of the first pressing ("virgin" is the result of the second) and therefore has more flavour and better quality: this is what we strongly recommend you to use when cooking.

No sirt menu would be complete without red wine, one of the cornerstones of the diet. It contains the activators of resveratrol and piceatannol sirtuins, which probably explain the longevity and slenderness associated with the traditional french way of life, and which are at the origin of the enthusiasm unleashed by sirt foods.

Of course, wine contains alcohol, so it should be consumed in moderation. Fortunately, resveratrol can withstand heat well, and therefore can be used in the kitchen. Pinot noir is many people's favourite grape variety because it contains much more resveratrol than most of the others.

On the sixth day, you will assume 2 green sirt juices and 2 solid meals (normal or vegan).

Drink the juices at different times of the day (for example, the first in the morning as soon as you wake up or in the middle of the morning, the second in the middle of the afternoon) and choose the normal or vegan dishes: super sirt salad and grilled beef fillet with red wine sauce, onion rings, garlic curly kale and roasted potatoes with aromatic herbs or super lentil sirt salad (vegan dish) and mole sauce of red beans with roasted potato (vegan dish).

Sunday: 2 green juices | breakfast: a bowl of sirt muesli + a cup of green juice | lunch: sirt food | snack: a cup of green juice | dinner: sirt food

The seventh day is the last of phase 1 of the diet. Instead of considering it as an end, see it as a beginning, because you are about to embark on a new life, in which sirt foods will play a central role in your nutrition. Today's menu is a perfect example of how easy it is to integrate them in abundance into your daily diet. Just take your favourite dishes and, with a pinch of creativity, you will turn them into a sirt banquet.

Walnuts are excellent sirt food because they contradict current opinions. They have high-fat content and many calories, yet it has been shown that they contribute to reducing weight and metabolic diseases, all thanks to the activation of sirtuins. They are also a versatile ingredient, excellent in baked dishes, in salads and as a snack, alone.

Pesto is becoming an irreplaceable ingredient in the kitchen because it is tasty and allows you to give personality to even the simplest dishes. The traditional one is made with basil and pine nuts, but you can try an alternative one with parsley and walnuts. The result is delicious and rich in sirt foods.

We can apply the same reasoning to an easy-to-prepare dish, such as an omelette. The dish has to be the typical recipe appreciated by the whole family, and simple to transform into a sirt dish with a few little tricks. In our recipe, we use bacon. Why? Simply because it fits perfectly. The sirtfood diet tells us what to include, not what to exclude, and this allows us to change our long-term eating habits. After all, isn't that the secret to not getting back the lost pounds and staying healthy?

On the seventh day, you will assume 2 green sirt juices; 2 solid meals (normal or vegan).

Drink the juices at different times of the day (for example the first in the morning as soon as you wake up or in the middle of the morning, the second in the middle of the afternoon) and choose the normal or vegan dishes.

During the second phase, there are no calorie restrictions but indications on which sirt foods must be eaten to consolidate weight loss and not run the risk of getting the lost kilos back.

The procedure of the sirtfood diet

The sirt food diet consists of three phases: in phase one, the body is relieved as with a gentle fast. In the second phase, you lose pounds; in the third phase, you keep the desired weight.

Sometimes two phases are spoken of, in which case the first phase consists of phase 1 and 2.

You can repeat these three phases as often as you want to lose weight. However, we recommend that you continue to "sirtify" your diet after these phases are complete by regularly including sirt foods in your meals. We also recommend that you continue drinking green juice or smoothies every day.

The 3 phases of the sirtfood diet:

- Phase 1: the first phase is the reprogramming of the metabolism to "lean". This works, for example, with sirtuin-rich green juices that detoxify the body. It lasts for three days. This means 1,000 calories per day in the form of 3 juices and 1 main meal.
- Phase 2: the calorie intake is increased to 1,500 calories. It lasts for four days. There are now 2 green juices and 2 main meals per day.
- Phase 3: serves to stabilise the new weight. In the third or "maintenance" phase, everything is allowed as long as you have as many sirt foods on the menu as possible and eat about 1800 calories. It lasts for two weeks. There are 1 green juice and 3 main meals per day.

Meal plan for three weeks

Phase 1, day 1-3:

In the first three days, you only consume 1,000kcal at a time. To be consumed:

· 3x green sirtfood juice · 1X main meal

Phase 2, day 4-7:

In the next four days, you will reach 1.500kcal. This is achieved by

· 2X green sirtfood juice · 2X main meal

During the introductory phase, you should drink water, green tea and black coffee.

Phase 3, day 8-21:

The second phase then lasts 14 days. There is also a fixed plan here, based on which there are:

· 1X green sirtfood juice · 3x main meal · 1-2X snacks

You should drink the juice first, about 30 minutes before breakfast. The dinner should be taken until 7 pm if possible. You should drink water, green tea or black coffee. Black or white tea is also fine. Red wine is also allowed, but not more than two to three glasses per week, otherwise the fat will be stored again.

Day 1
-3x green sirtfood juice
-1X main meal

Day 2
-3x green sirtfood juice
-1X main meal

Day 3
-3x green sirtfood juice
-1X main meal

Day 4
-2X green sirtfood juice
-2X main meal

Day 5
-2X green sirtfood juice
-2X main meal

Day 6
-2X green sirtfood juice
-2X main meal

Day 7
-2X green sirtfood juice -2X main meal

Day 8
-1X green sirtfood juice
-3x main meal

Day 9
-1X green sirtfood juice
-3x main meal

Day 10
-1X green sirtfood juice
-3x main meal

Day 11
-1X green sirtfood juice
-3x main meal

Day 12
-1X green sirtfood juice
-3x main meal

Day 13
-1X green sirtfood juice
-3x main meal

Day 14
-1X green sirtfood juice
-3x main meal

Day 15
-1X green sirtfood juice
-3x main meal

Day 16
-1X green sirtfood juice
-3x main meal

Day 17
-1X green sirtfood juice
-3x main meal

Day 18
-1X green sirtfood juice
-3x main meal

Day 19
-1X green sirtfood juice
-3x main meal

Day 20
-1X green sirtfood juice
-3x main meal

Day 21
-1X green sirtfood juice
-3x main meal

Expectations for phase 1

In the first seven days of the diet, you should anticipate losing up to 7 lbs. The wording of this sentence is important – you may lose 7 lbs, but many people don't see such dramatic changes.

Bear in mind that the sirtfood diet may also result in a gain in muscle mass, another reason why the 7 lbs loss may not be achieved. Instead of the precise weight value, it's better to look for signs that your body is changing. Do your clothes fit better? Do you feel better? Has your skin improved?

Looking for other signs of the diet is also important because the sirtfood diet isn't just a weight loss scheme – it is intended to promote overall body health, so you should anticipate overall improvements. The authors of the sirtfood diet even go so far as to suggest that you can purchase some basic health measurement tools from your local pharmacies, such as a blood pressure monitor or blood sugar monitor to check for changes.

Finally, you need to change your outlook. The sirtfood diet is intended to replace your normal eating habits eventually, and so you need to go into the diet with a willingness and adaptivity to generate a long-term change.

It is recommended that you space your three juices out between the day, instead of consuming them in rapid succession. You should avoid drinking any of the juices any hour before or after your main meal.

It is also suggested that you should also not consume any of your juices, or your main meal, after 7 pm. This is advised due to our natural circadian rhythms (or our 'body clock') and how they affect our body. Generally speaking, our body wants to prepare and burn energy in the morning, while store and retain energy during the evening. Therefore if you eat later atnight, you have a higher chance of the energy in your food being stored asfat.

In fact, some evidence also supports the idea that sirtuins can enhance and support the circadian rhythm, increasing the amount of energy you burn in the morning.

On top of this, it is also advised that you don't force yourself to eat your meal or consume your juices if you feel too full. Surprisingly, although you are at a notable calorie deficit during the first few days, many people report that they don't feel hungry. In fact, the contrast is true, with people often claiming they are completely stuffed. Owing to this, if you can't consume all your intake of the first few days, don't worry.

You should also feel free to drink non-calorie fluids. While this technically does include calorie-free fizzy drinks, the authors of the diet promote green tea, black coffee and of course, water, as good choices. One surprising finding is that small doses of lemon juice can prove helpful in increasing sirtuin absorption, so consider add a dash to your water or greentea.

Note that only black coffee is heartily recommended, with milk, sugar and sweeteners diminishing the sirtuin absorption and interfering with the calorie count. Another caveat is that you shouldn't change your coffee consumption too much from your regular habits. A sudden drop in consumption will make you feel awful; a sharp increase will make you feel jittery. Change your coffee habits gradually.

Day-by-day breakdown

Day 1, 2 & 3 you should be aware of the formula by now – three green juices taken in the morning, midday and evening with a main meal in between. You can select any of the main meals covered in the recipe section.

Additionally, you can also have 20g of dark chocolate, as long as the chocolate is at least 85% cocoa solids. There's also a process called dutch processing which is applied to chocolate that diminishes the nutritional value. As a result, you should try to avoid certain brands that use dutch processing by choosing alternative brands.

Day 4, 5, 6 & 7. Your calorie count gets increased to 1,500, and you drop one of the green juices for a second main meal. You also, unfortunately, drop the chocolate. Ensure that you are not repetitive with your selection of meals – you need variety and you shouldn't have needed to repeat a meal, as of yet.

How to jumpstart your sirtfood diet?

Fat burning, increasing muscles, and better cellular fitness – these are the guaranteed results of the sirtfood diet.

Being healthy and losing weight is an everyday choice. You have to take those first baby steps and see how it can change you and your life.

If you want to reap the fantastic results of sirtfoods, here are some suggested ways to jumpstart your diet:

Safety first - before starting any particular diet or regimen, consult your healthcare provider, especially if you have existing illnesses. This will ensure that the diet will not sabotage any medications that you might be taking or harm your health. Do not worry; the sirtfood diet is safe.

Knowledge is power - this diet is still brand new, but there is still a good amount of information available and more upcoming since this diet is fast gaining popularity. Also, you can search the internet for recipes, food alternatives, nutrient content and more.

Follow the guidelines - sirtfood is guaranteed to bring results, if and only if you carefully follow the diet guide and suggested food.

Help yourself - aside from following what is allowed in the food prog; you can start by eliminating processed and starchy food from your normal diet. Stop eating junk! This will fast track the result of sirtfood diet.

Start a physical activity - sirtfood diet can indeed burn those fats and build muscle, but I recommend that you start adding physical activities to your daily routine. A 30-minute walk a day would do wonders to your body and will also fast track the results. Also, there are many wonderful effects when exercising like preventing and combating health conditions, helping improve your mood, promoting better sleep, burning calories, giving you an energy boost and more.

Hit the supermarket - the sirtfood diet depends on certain foods. These foods were chosen because of their sirtuin-triggering ability. So if you do not follow the list, well, you won't see results. Do not worry, because I will be providing a list of suggested foods; plus there are no overly expensive type of foods, and you can find it readily available almost anywhere (you might even already have some lurking in your fridge).

Be ready with the initial "restrictions" - of course, if you want to see different results, you have to "sacrifice" a little to achieve the full benefits of the sirtfood diet. But don't worry, the first three days are only the hardest ones for this diet since there will be calorie restrictions involved, but rest assured that it will become easier each day. Although for others who tried the diet, the restrictions set was not that hard for them, the reason is careful planning of meals. You will not go hungry with this diet if you choose wisely.

Involve a diet partner - this diet could also greatly benefit your family, partner or friends (not only for overweight individuals), plus it is easier when you have an accountability partner to remind you, share recipes with or even cook dishes with.

Document your progress - you can start by taking "before" pictures and take necessary body measurements. You could also keep a food diary so that you can watch your food intake. Observe the changes in your body with each week or phase. You can also have a set of goals to push you further to continue with the diet.

Be kind to yourself - do not set too high expectations. Yes, some can easily lose 7lbs in a week, but remember that our bodies are not all the same; and of course, your level of commitment will also count. Other variables could be adding an exercise regimen in the diet plan, which could make the losing weight process faster.

Chapter 4: What's a "skinny gene"?

The skinny gene-diet is not difficult to follow and is divided into two phases. The first phase lasts 7 days and is more restrictive and difficult, especially for the first 3 days. To be able to lose 3 kg per week as promised by this diet, it is advisable, initially, not to exceed 1,000 calories per day during the first 3 days, drinking 3 green juices based on sirtuin-rich foods and eating only one solid meal of your choice, prepared using the ingredients indicated above.

From the 4th to the 7th day, instead, you can ingest 1,500 calories per day by consuming three green juices and two solid meals composed of foods rich in sirtuins.

The sirtfood diet also called the skinny gene-diet, is the result of the studies of the two nutritionists Aidan Goggins and Glenn Matten. Their food prog, published in a volume that explains its principles and functioning, has attracted the attention of VIPs and athletes. Its effectiveness is based on the consumption of foods that stimulate sirtuins. As the creators of the diet of the moment explain, it is a family of genes present in each of us. They affect the ability to burn fat in addition to mood and the mechanisms that regulate longevity. It is no coincidence that they are also called "super metabolic regulators." Recent studies have shown that several foods can stimulate sirtuins. Their consumption would, therefore, allow them to activate the metabolism and lose weight without having to undergo extremediets.

What makes the sirtfood diet different from the others is its "inclusion" philosophy. In fact, it is not based on the total or partial exclusion of some foods from your diet. Rather, it suggests which foods should be added to lose weight more easily. In this way, you will no longer have to undergo excessive deprivation or exhausting willpower. And you won't have to resort to expensive supplements or products with mysterious components. By eating a balanced diet and supporting it, if desired, with proper physical activity, according to the two nutritionists, you can lose about 3.5kg in a week.

Sirt foods are particularly rich in special nutrients, capable of activating the same genes of thinness stimulated by fasting. These genes are sirtuins. They became famous thanks to an important study conducted in 2003, during which scientists analysed a particular substance, resveratrol, present in the peel of black grapes, red wine, and yeast, which would produce the same effects of calorie restriction without need to decrease your daily calories intake. Later, researchers found that other substances in red wine had a similar effect, which would explain the benefits of consuming this drink and why those who consume it get less fat.

This naturally stimulated the search for other foods containing a high concentration of these nutrients, capable of producing such a beneficial effect on the body, and studies gradually discovered several. If some are almost unknown, such as lovage, an herb that is by now very littleused in cooking, the great majority is represented by well-known and widely used foods, such as extra virgin olive oil, red onions, parsley, chilli, kale, strawberries, capers, tofu, cocoa, green tea, and even coffee.

After the discovery in 2003, the enthusiasm for the benefits of sort's food skyrocketed. Studies revealed that these foods don't just mimic the effects of calorie restriction. They also act as super regulators of the entire metabolism: they burn fat, increase muscle mass, and improve the health of our cells. The world of medical research was close to the most important nutritional discovery of the century. Unfortunately, a mistake was made: the pharmaceutical industry invested hundreds of millions of pounds in an attempt to turn sirt foods into a sort of miracle pill, and the diet took a back seat. The sirtfood diet, however, does not share this pharmaceutical approach, which seeks (so far without result) to concentrate the benefits of these complex nutrients of plant origin into a single drug. Instead of waiting for the pharmaceutical industry to transform the nutrients of the foods we eat into a miraculous product (which may not work anyway), the sirtfood diet consists of eating these substances in their natural form that of food, to take full advantage of them. This is the basis of the pilot experiment of the sirtfood diet, with which the creators intended to create a diet containing the richest sources of sirt foods and observe their effects.

During their studies, Glen Matten and Aidan Goggins discovered that the best sirt foods are consumed regularly by populations who boast the lowest incidence of diseases and obesity in the world.

The Kuna Indians, in the American continent, seem immune from hypertension and with very low levels of obesity, diabetes, cancer, and early death thanks to the intake of cocoa, excellent sirt food. In Okinawa, Japan, sirt food, dry physique, and longevity go hand in hand. In India, the passion for spicy foods, especially turmeric, gives good results in the fight against cancer. And in the traditional Mediterranean diet, which the rest of the western world envies, obesity is contained, and chronic diseases are the exception, not the norm. extra virgin olive oil, wild green leafy vegetables, dried fruit, berries, red wine, dates, and aromatic herbs are all effective sirt foods, and they are all present in the Mediterranean diet. The scientific world has had to surrender to the evidence: it seems that the Mediterranean diet is more effective than reducing calories to lose weight and more effective than drugs to eliminate diseases.

Although sirt foods are not a mainstay of nutrition in most of the western world today, the situation was quite different in the past. They were a basic element, and if many have become rare and others have even disappeared, it is definitely possible to reverse the course of this.

The good news is that you don't have to be a top athlete, and not even sporty, to enjoy the same benefits. We took advantage of everything we learned about sirt foods thanks to the pilot study by kx and the work done with sportsmen, and we adapted it to create a diet suitable for anyone who wants to lose weight while improving health.

It is not necessary to practice unsustainable fasting or to undergo endless sessions in the gym (although, of course, practising a little physical activity would be good for you). It is not an expensive diet, nor will it waste your time, and all the foods recommended in the diet are readily available. The only accessory you will need is an extractor or centrifuge. Unlike other diets, which tell you what to eliminate, this diet tells you what to eat.

Generally, you can eat foods that are high in protein and low in fat. Among the meat-based recipes, you can choose, for example, chicken with red onion and black cabbage, turkey with cauliflower couscous, turkey escalope with capers and parsley. For fish dishes, sautéed salmon fillet, sautéed prawns, or baked marinated cod are fine.

Recipes of side dishes, light and tasty, can be prepared with beans, lentils, aubergines cut into wedges, and cooked in the oven, Walldorf salad, or red onions. And as for dessert, you can eat delicious and healthy strawberries, with a very high content of sirtuins. Plus, remember that 15-20g of dark chocolate are allowed every day.

The green juice is an important part of the diet, because it has the ability to cleanse and detoxify, and will be the protagonist in the first week of the sirt prog.

Sirt foods are particularly rich in special nutrients of plant origin recently discovered, which, stimulated by fasting, activate the genes of thinness.

The foods suggested in the sirtfood diet are fresh, genuine and easily available, such as extra virgin olive oil, dark chocolate, citrus fruits, strawberries, apples, cabbage, celery, spinach, buckwheat, blueberries, nuts, soya beans, rocket salad, red onion, coffee, green tea**, red wine, chilli pepper***, tofu, turmeric, and dates.

In addition, combined with each other or with other foods, they allow you to create very tasty dishes.

Sirtuins filled ingredients

Cocoa

Yes, to chocolate, but not any type! It must be dark chocolate and present at least 85% of cocoa. Useful above all to appease hunger, therefore mostly used as a snack.

Lindt excellence 85%, which retains a good percentage of flavonoids, and Rowntree's cocoa powder are the most highly recommended.

Chilli pepper***

To make your dishes spicier, use bird's eye chilli (also called Thai chilli), very rich in sirtuin. You can use it at least three times a week.

Warning! Compared to normal chilli, the bird's eye is much spicier; to get used to it, in the beginning, use only half of what is indicated in the recipe, eliminating the seeds, which are very spicy.

Coffee

You can drink 3-4 cups of coffee a day being careful not to overdo it with sugar, and avoid adding milk.

Green tea**

Known because it is so good for our body, green tea contributes to the loss of fat, preserving your muscles. Choose the matcha variety and drink it with the addition of a little lemon juice, which increases the absorption of the nourishing activators of sirtuins.

Red wine

The research that gave rise to the sirtfood diet started with red wine. The first sirt slimming element discovered, in fact, is resveratrol, present in black grape's skin and red wine. It appears that this nutrient attacks fat cells. In addition, red wine contains piceatannol, associated with longevity.

Kale

Kale is a suitable food for every diet. It is cheap and easy to find. It contains in large quantities two nutrients that activate sirtuins: kaempferol and quercetin, which act in synergy to prevent the formation of fat.

Buckwheat

This "pseudo-cereal" is very popular in Japan and is a nutritious and highly satiating food, properties on which this type of nutrition focuses. So yes, to seeds, flakes, and buckwheat pasta.

Celery

The nutritive parts of celery, used for millennia, also as a medicinal plant, are the heart and the leaves: here, in fact, the activators of the sirtuins are contained, which are apigenin and luteolin. A tip: if you can, choose the green one instead of the white one.

Medjoul dates

Although dates are composed of 66% sugar, they also contain "good" polyphenols that activate sirtuins. So, unlike normal sugars, date nutrients do not increase the amount of glucose in the blood, but their consumption seems instead associated with a lower incidence of diabetes and heart disease. However, always remember to eat them in moderation!

Capers

The caper plant is widespread in Mediterranean countries, and its fruits are highly appreciated for their "concentrate of taste" capable of reviving even the most anonymous dishes. Taste aside, capers are also very rich in active-sirtuin nutrients, such as kaempferol and quercetin.

Extra virgin olive oil

Good and healthy, the extra virgin olive oil, obtained from the first pressing of the olives, is a perfect seasoning and tastes very good both on vegetables and on bread! Rich in polyphenols, vitamin-e and "good" fatty acids, it will be your heart and youth's best friend, thanks to its antioxidant properties.

Rocket salad

Arugula is a vegetable rich in nutrients that activate the metabolism, such as quercetin and kaempferol. Its peppery and decisive flavour can embellish many recipes, and it especially goes with olive oil.

A curiosity: they began to cultivate it for the first time in ancient Rome, where it seems it was very appreciated for its aphrodisiac qualities.

Parsley

It is a basic ingredient to enrich practically any dish and a lot of sauces. It tastes fresh and is used to relieve itching and toothache. The sirtfood diet appreciates it above all because it is one of the foods with the highest concentration of apigenin, an activator of sirtuins.

Red chicory

It can be consumed within this diet in large quantities, both alone and accompanied by other sirt foods. A greedy idea? Caramelized red chicory salad with celery leaves.

Soy

In addition to its beneficial properties, associated with the activating action of daidzein and formononetin, soy has an unmistakable flavour that makes every dish tastier.

Soy sauce, soy yoghurt, and miso, a traditional Japanese dish based on salt-fermented soybeans, are all amazing. Red (saltier) and brown miso, are the most suitable qualities to prepare sirt recipes

Red onion

Tasty and rich in quercetin, which activates the metabolism. It is important to peel it and consume it raw to keep the nutrients active so that they can act better on sirtuins.

Strawberries

They have few sugars, are delicious and will also make you lose weight because they are the main source of fisetin, a sirtuin activator.

Walnuts

They are rich in fats and very caloric, yet, according to sirt nutritionists, this food should promote weight loss by also fighting metabolic diseases. In addition, walnuts contain a lot of minerals, which are extremely useful for the body, such as magnesium, zinc, copper, calcium, and iron. An idea for a first course? Try an alternative pesto with walnuts and parsley.

Supplements

In the presence of food deficiencies, it may be appropriate to restore the body's balance by providing it with an extra dose of those nutrients that are missing or are in short supply in our everyday diet. However, remember that supplements shouldn't be eaten "for fun", so it is always advisable to seek medical advice before taking any product, even if it is as natural as it comes

What does the sirtfood diet include?

Stage 1 of the sirtfood diet is the hyper-achievement stage, a 7-day plan demonstrated to help lose 7lbs. During the initial three days, calorie admission is confined to 1,000 calories for every day, comprising of three sirtfood green juices, in addition to one full dinner rich in sirtfoods. On days four to seven, calorie consumption increments to 1,500 calories, involving two sirtfood-rich green juices and two sirtfood-rich suppers.

Stage 2 is a 14-day upkeep stage, where weight loss proceeds consistently. It's tied in with pressing the diet brimming with an abundance of sirtfoods which is accomplished by eating three adjusted sirtfood-rich dinners day by day, alongside a 'support' sirtfood green juice.

In our sirtfood diet, preliminary members lost a great 7lbs over the underlying 7 days remembering increments for muscle and muscle work. This emotional impact on fat-consuming, while advancing muscle, is one reason that our sirtfood-based diet has gotten so mainstream with anybody needing to get slender and fit as a fiddle, much the same as the world-class competitors and models who have supported along these lines of eating. Alongside fat consuming, sirtfoods additionally have the extraordinary capacity to normally satisfy hunger making them the ideal answer for accomplishing a sound weight and continuing it long haul.

Be that as it may, to consider it absolutely as a weight loss diet is to overlook the main issue. This is a diet that has as a lot to do with health as waistlines. Expanded vitality, more clear skin, feeling alarm progressively, and better rest is the charming 'symptoms' from along these lines of eating. Now and again, the advantages are much progressively exceptional, remembering situations where following the diet for the more drawn out term has turned around metabolic ailments. Such is their wellbeing improving impacts that reviews demonstrate them to be all the more dominant then physician endorsed medicates in forestalling constant malady, with benefits in diabetes, coronary illness and Alzheimer's to give some examples. It's no big surprise that it is entrenched that the way of life eating the most sirtfoods have been the least fatty and most beneficial on the planet.

The primary concern is clear: if you need to accomplish a progressively fiery, less fatty and more advantageous body, and establish the frameworks for lifelong wellbeing and protection from sickness, then the sirtfood diet is for you.

Here at the international food information council foundation, we ramble about trend diets. For the most part, we're exposing them and advancing a fair eating arrangement with space for guilty pleasures and festivities. Now and then the diets we talk about depend on some strong sustenance rules, and others we can't accept truly exist. This next diet we're going to discuss falls into the last class. The most recent on the diet scene is the sirtfood diet, and we're here to disclose to you why you needn't bother with that sort of limitation in your life: it's not science-based or practical.

Chapter 5: Cancer preventing superfoods

The best thing about this diet is that you are not always forced to starve yourself. Phase 1 and phase 2 can be repeated from time to time to lose fat if necessary. For someone, it might be essential to repeat them every three months, while for someone other people, it will be enough to repeat it once a year. The rest of the time, you are free to live your life, skinnier, and healthier than before, continuing to enjoy the benefits of a diet rich in sirt foods. In fact, these foods have a universal application and can be incorporated in any type of dietary regime: vegan, gluten-free, low in carbohydrates, intermittent fasting, and so on. Incorporating significant quantities of sirt foods will enhance the weight loss and health benefits of all those approaches.

The secret of success is to achieve results that will last a lifetime, and the sirtfood diet is truly exceptional in that sense. When you will have assimilated the cornerstones of a balanced diet and the correct use of supplements, and you have discovered the practical tips to consume even more sirt foods, you will be ready to benefit from them for the rest of your life.

Here is a list of the benefits of the sirtfood diet: promotes fat loss, not muscle loss; you will not regain weight after the end of the diet; you will look better; you will feel better, and you will have more energy; you will avoid fasting and feeling hungry; you will not have to undergo exhausting physical exercises; this diet promotes a longer, healthier life and keeps diseases away.

The benefits of the sirtfood diet are many, besides obviously that of slimming. Activators of sirtuins would lead to a noticeable muscle building, decreased appetite, and improved memory. In addition, the sirtfood diet normalizes the level of sugar in the blood and is able to cleanse the cells from the accumulation of harmful free radicals.

The sirtfood diet depends on a newfound gathering of nourishments called sirtfoods. These miracle nourishments can initiate an amazing reusing process in the body that gets out cell waste and consumes fat. They do this by enacting our sirtuin qualities – otherwise called our "thin" qualities. These are similar qualities that are actuated by exercise and fasting.

Top sirtfoods incorporate kale, rocket, parsley, red onions, strawberries, pecans, additional virgin olive oil, cocoa, curry flavours, green tea and espresso (truly, espresso!). As opposed to past advanced diets where the emphasis is on removing nourishments, with sirtfoods, the advantages are harvested through eating.

Chapter 6: Breakfast

Cranberry quinoa breakfast

Preparation time: 10 minutes| Cooking time: 20 minutes| Servings: 2

Ingredients:

½ cup quinoa

1 cup milk

2-3 tbsp honey, optional

1 tsp cinnamon

½ tsp vanilla

1 tsp ground flaxseed

2 tbsp walnuts or almonds, chopped

2 tbsp dried cranberries

Directions:

Rinse quinoa and drain.

Combine milk, quinoa and flaxseed into a saucepan.

Bring to a boil, add in cinnamon and vanilla and simmer for about 15 minutes.

When done, place a portion of the quinoa into a bowl, drizzle with honey, and top with cranberries and crushed walnuts.

Green omelet

Preparation time: 10 minutes| Cooking time: 30 minutes| Servings: 2

Ingredients:

2 large eggs, at room temperature

1 shallot, peeled and chopped

Handful arugula

3 sprigs of parsley, chopped

1 tsp extra virgin olive oil

Salt and black pepper

Directions:

Beat the eggs in a small bowl and set aside.

Sauté the shallot for 5 minutes with a bit of the oil, on low-medium heat.

Pour the eggs in the pans, stirring the mixture for just a second.

The eggs on medium heat, and tip the pan just enough to let the loose egg run underneath after about one minute on the burner.

Add the greens, herbs, and the seasonings to the top side as it is still soft.

Tip: you do not even have to flip it, as you can just cook the egg slowly egg as is well (being careful as to not burn).

Tip: Another option is to put it into an oven to broil for 3-5 minutes (checking to make sure it is only until it is golden but burned).

Berry oat breakfast cobbler

Preparation time: 10 minutes | Cooking time: 40 minutes | Servings: 2

Ingredients:

2 cups of oats/flakes that are ready without cooking

1 cup of blackcurrants without the stems

1 tsp of honey (or ¼ tsp of raw sugar)

½ cup of water (add more or less by testing the pan)

1 cup of plain yoghurt (or soy orcoconut)

Directions:

Boil the berries, honey and water and then turn it down on low.

Put in a glass container in a refrigerator until it is cool and set (about 30 minutes or more)

When ready to eat, scoop the berries on top of the oats and yoghurt.

Serve immediately.

Pancakes with apples and blackcurrants

Preparation time: 10 minutes | Cooking time: 20 minutes | Servings: 2

Ingredients:

2 apples, cut into small chunks

2 cups of quick cooking oats

1 cup flour of your choice

1 tsp baking powder

2 tbsp raw sugar, coconut sugar, or 2 tbsp honey that is warm and easy todistribute

2 egg whites

1 ¼ cups of milk (or soy/rice/coconut)

2 tsp extra virgin olive oil

A dash of salt

For the berry topping:

1 cup blackcurrants, washed and stalks removed

3 tbsp Water (may use less)

2 tbsp Sugar (see above for types)

Directions:

Place the ingredients for the topping in a small pot simmer, stirring frequently for about 10 minutes until it cooks down and the juices are released.

Take the dry ingredients and mix in a bowl.

After, add the apples and the milk a bit at a time (you may not use it all), until it is a batter.

Stiffly whisk the egg whites and then gently mix them into the pancake batter.

Set aside in the refrigerator.

Pour a one quarter of the oil onto a flat pan or flat griddle, and when hot, pour some of the batter into it in a pancake shape.

When the pancakes start to have golden brown edges and form air bubbles, they may be ready to be gently flipped.

Test to be sure the bottom can life away from the pan before actually flipping.

Repeat for the next three pancakes.

Top each pancake with the berries.

Berry quinoa and chia seed breakfast

Preparation time: 5 minutes | Cooking time: 30 minutes| Servings: 3

Ingredients:

½ cup quinoa

1½ cups milk

2 tbsp chia seeds

¼ cup fresh blueberries or raspberries

2 tbsp pistachios, silvered

Directions:

Combine quinoa and chia seeds with milk and bring to a boil.

Cover, reduce heat and simmer for 15 minutes.

When ready, serve into bowls and top with fresh berries and pistachios.

Sirtfood truffle bites

Preparation time: 10 minutes | Cooking time: 20 minutes |Servings: 2

Ingredients:

1 cup walnuts

¾ cup of Medjool dates, pitted

½ cup of dark chocolate broken into pieces; or cocoa nibs

2 heaping tbsp of cacao powder

½ cup of dried coconut

1 tbsp ground turmeric

1 tbsp extra virgin olive oil, or coconut oil (preferred)

1 tsp vanilla extract, or a vanilla pod, scraped

1 dash of cayenne pepper

1 dash sea salt (up to 1/8 tsp)

2 tbsp water if needed

Directions:

Pulse in a food processor the walnuts and chocolate until finely pulverized.

Gently blend solid ingredients next and the vanilla.

Make a dough.

Make rolled balls out of the dough.

Add water a few drops at a time only if it is necessary.

Do not use too much water, or you will have to go and add more of the other ingredients to compensate.

Refrigerate.

Store for up to a week.

Take them with you to work or when travelling for a quick pick-me-up as well as to quell a sweet tooth.

Spicy kale chips

Preparation time: 10 minutes | Cooking time: 30 minutes | Servings: 2

Ingredients:

1 large head of curly kale, wash, dry and pulled from stem 1 tbsp extra virgin olive oil

Minced parsley

Squeeze of lemon juice

Cayenne pepper (just a pinch)

Dash of soy sauce

Directions:

In a large bowl, rip the kale from the stem into palm sized pieces.

Sprinkle the minced parsley, olive oil, soy sauce, a squeeze of the lemon juice and a very small pinch of the cayenne powder.

Toss with a set if tongs or salad forks, and make sure to coat all of the leaves.

If you have a dehydrator, turn it on to 118F, spread out the kale on a dehydrator sheet, and leave in there for about 2 hours.

If you are cooking them, place parchment paper on top of a cookie sheet.

Lay the bed of kale and separate it a bit to make sure the kale is evenly toasted.

Cook for 10-15 minutes maximum at 250F.

Sweet and savory guacamole

Preparation time: 10 minutes | Cooking time: 20 minutes | Servings: 2

Ingredients:

2 large avocados, pitted and scooped

2 Medjool dates, pitted and chopped into small pieces

½ cup cherry tomatoes, cut into halves

5 sprigs of parsley, chopped

¼ cup of arugula, chopped

5 sticks of celery, washed, cut into sticks for dipping

Juice from ¼ lime

Dash of sea salt

Directions:

Mash the avocado in a bowl, sprinkle salt, and squeeze of the lime juice.

Fold in the tomatoes, dates, herbs and greens.

Scoop with celery sticks, and enjoy!

Thai nut mix

Preparation time: 10 minutes | Cooking time: 20 minutes | Servings: 2

Ingredients:

½ cup walnuts

½ cup coconut flakes

½ tsp soy sauce

1 tsp honey

1 pinch of cayenne pepper

1 dash of lime juice

Directions:

Add the above ingredients to a bowl, toss the nuts to coat, and place on a baking sheet, lined with parchment paper.

Cook at 250F for 15-20 minutes, checking as not to burn, but lightly toasted.

Remove from oven.

Cool first before eating.

Berry yoghurt freeze

Preparation time: 10 minutes | Cooking time: 25 minutes | Servings: 2

Ingredients:

2 cups plain yoghurt (Greek, soy or coconut)

½ cup sliced strawberries

½ cup blackberries

1 tsp honey (warmed)

½ tsp chocolate powder

Directions:

Blend all of the above ingredients until creamy in a bowl.

Place into two glass or in metal bowls that are freezer-safe, and put into the freezer for 1 hour.

Remove and thaw just slightly so that it is soft enough to eat with a spoon.

Buckwheat pita bread

Preparation time: 10 minutes | Cooking time: 20 minutes | Servings: 2

Ingredients:

1 x 8g packet dried yeast

Polenta for dusting

3 tbsp of olive oil

375ml lukewarm water

500g buckwheat flour

1 tsp of sea salt

Directions:

Combine the yeast and water and let the mixture activate (approximately 10 to 15 minutes).

Combine the buckwheat flour, olive oil, salt and add in the yeast mixture.

Knead it slowly until you make dough.

Cover and place in a warm spot for about an hour (to rise).

Evenly divide the dough into six pieces.

Take a piece, shape it to a flat disc, and then place it in between 2 sheets of baking paper.

Carefully roll out the dough into a ¼-inch thick round pita shapes.

Using a fork, pierce the dough a couple of times and lightly dust it with the polenta.

Heat a 10-inch cast iron and smear it with olive oil.

Cook the bread on one side until puffy then do the same with the other side.

Fill up with desired vegetables and meat and serve immediately.

Alternatively, you could wrap it in foil, place in the fridge, and reheat in the oven the next day.

Smoked salmon omelette

Preparation time: 10 minutes | Cooking time: 10 minutes | Servings: 2

Ingredients:

10g of chopped rocket

100g smoked salmon, sliced

1 tsp of extra virgin olive oil

½ tsp of capers

2 medium eggs

1 tsp of chopped parsley

Directions:

Crack the eggs into a bowl, and whisk them well.

Add the capers, parsley, rocket, and salmon and heat oil in a non-stick pan until hot but not smoking.

Add the egg mixture into the pan andmove it around the pan using a spatula.

Reduce the heat to low and let the omelet cook.

Slide the spatula under the omelette, fold it up in half, and serve.

Pancakes with blackcurrant compote

Preparation time: 10 minutes | Cooking time: 30 minutes | Servings: 2

Ingredients:

2 tsp of light olive oil

125g of plain flour

75g of porridge oats

2 apples (peeled, cored and cut into tiny pieces)

1 tsp of baking powder

2 egg whites

Pinch of salt

300ml semi-skimmed milk

2 tbsp of caster sugar

For the compote:

120g blackcurrants, washed and stalks removed

3 tbsp of water

2 tbsp of caster sugar

Directions:

Make the compote first.

Place the blackcurrants, water, and sugar in a small pan.

Bring it to a simmer and let it cook for 10 to 15 minutes.

Place oats, caster sugar, baking powder, flour, and salt in a large bowl and stir well.

Add in the apple then the milk a little at a time as you whisk until you have a smooth batter.

Whisk the egg whites into stiff peaks and fold into the pancake batter.

Transfer the ready batter to a jug.

In a frying pan, placed on medium high heat, heat ½ tsp of oil and add in approximately a quarter of the batter.

Let it cook on both sides until it turns golden brown.

Remove when ready then repeat to make four pancakes.

Drizzle the blackcurrant compote over the pancakes and serve.

Chocolate chips granola

Preparation time: 10 minutes | Cooking time: 30 minutes | Servings: 2

Ingredients: 2 tbsp of rice malt syrup

20g of butter 200g of jumbo oats

60g of good-quality (70%) dark chocolate chips 3 tbsp of light olive oil

1 tbsp of dark brown sugar

50g of roughly chopped pecans

Directions:

Preheat your oven to 160°c.

Use baking parchment or silicone sheet to line a large baking tray.

Add the pecans and oats into a large bowl and mix.

Add butter, olive oil, rice malt syrup, and brown sugar to a small pan and gently heat until the butter melts and the syrup and sugar dissolves (do not allow to boil).

Drizzle the syrup over the oats and stir thoroughly until the oats are fully coated.

Distribute granola all over the baking tray and leave clumps of with a bit of spacing instead of an even spread.

Allow to bake in the oven until you see a tinge of golden brown on the edges (about 20 minutes).

Remove them and allow to cool.

Once cooled, break up the bigger lumps and mix in chocolate chips.

Serve and enjoy.

Scoop the remaining granola into an airtight jar.

It will keep for about 2 WEEks.

Breakfast scramble

Preparation time: 10 minutes | Cooking time: 20 minutes | Servings: 2

Ingredients:

A handful of button mushrooms, sliced thinly

1 tsp of mild curry powder

5g of parsley, chopped finely

½ bird's eye chilli, sliced thinly

1 tsp of ground turmeric

2 eggs

1 tsp of extra virgin olive oil

20g kale, chopped roughly

Optional-add seed mixture as toppings and rooster sauce for flavour

Directions:

Mix the curry powder and turmeric, and then add a little water until you have a light paste.

Steam the kale for about 2 to 3 minutes.

Place a frying pan over medium heat and heat the oil.

Fry the mushroom and chilli for 2 to 3 minutes until they start to soften and brown.

Add the paste, cook the eggs, and then serve.

Raspberry and blackcurrant jelly

Preparation time: 10 minutes | Cooking time: 25 minutes | Servings: 2

Ingredients:

100g of raspberries, washed

100g of blackcurrant (washed and stalks removed)

2 leaves of gelatin

300ml water

2 tbsp of granulated sugar

Directions:

Arrange the raspberries in 2 serving glasses or dishes.

Add cold water to a bowl and place the gelatin leaves in so they can soften.

In a small pan, add sugar, 100ml water, and the blackcurrant and boil.

Allow this to simmer for 5 minutes then remove from the heat.

Leave it for 2 minutes then take the gelatin leaves and squeeze out any excess water.

Add the leaves to the saucepan and stir until they fully dissolve.

Add in the rest of the water.

Pour the liquid in prepared dishes and refrigerate.

The jellies will be ready in about 3 to 4 hours overnight.

Strawberry buckwheat tabbouleh

Preparation time: 10 minutes | Cooking time: 20 minutes | Servings: 2

Ingredients:

65g of tomato

1 tbsp of ground turmeric

50g of buckwheat

1 tbsp of extra virgin olive oil

30g of parsley

100g of hulled strawberries

30g of rocket

80g of avocado

20g of red onions

1 tbsp of capers

Juice of ½ lemon

25G of Medjool dates, pitted

Dircctions:

Cook the buckwheat and the turmeric following the packet directions

Drain, and then set aside to let it cool.

Finely chop the avocado, parsley, red onion, tomato, dates, and capers and mix it with the cool buckwheat.

Slice strawberries and gently mix into the salad together with the lemon juice and oil.

Serve them on a bed of rocket.

Easy quinoa crackers

Preparation time: 10 minutes | Cooking time: 40 minutes | Servings: 2

Ingredients:

2 cups cooked quinoa

1 cup ground flaxseed

2 tbsp sesame seeds

1 tbsp honey 1 tsp salt

1 cup water

3 tbsp extra virgin olive oil

1 tsp garlic powder (optional)

½ tsp dried oregano (optional)

Directions:

Thoroughly mix together all ingredients in a large bowl.

Place the dough on a lined baking sheet and with wet hands, flatten the dough.

Slip the parchment off of the baking sheet, cover the length of the dough with plastic wrap and roll out the dough with a rolling pin to a ¼ inch thickness.

Bake at 350 f for 35 minutes or until the parchment paper easily pulls away and the dough is cooked but not crisp yet.

Flip the cracker over, gently remove the parchment paper and cut into squares.

Bake for another 35 minutes, or until the crackers are nice and crisp.

Granola-the sirt way

Preparation time: 10 minutes | Cooking time: 50 minutes | Servings: 2

Ingredients:

1 cup buckwheat puffs

1 cup buckwheat flakes (ready to eat type, but not whole buckwheat that needs to be cooked)

½ cup coconut flakes

½ cup Medjool dates, without pits, chopped into smaller, bite-sized pieces

1 cup of cacao nibs or very dark chocolate chips

½ cup walnuts, chopped

1 cup strawberries chopped and without stems

1 cup plain Greek, coconut or soy yoghurt.

Directions:

Mix, without yoghurt and strawberry toppings.

You can store for up to a week. Store in an airtight container.

Add toppings (even different berries or different yoghurt).

You can even use the berry toppings as you will learn how to make from other recipes.

Ginger prawn stir-fry

Preparation time: 10 minutes | Cooking time: 40 minutes | Servings: 2

Ingredients:

6 prawns or shrimp (peeled and deveined)

½ package of buckwheat noodles (called soba in Asian sections)

5-6 leaves of kale, chopped

1 cup of green beans, chopped

5g lovage or celery leaves

1 garlic clove, finely chopped

1 bird's eye chilli, finely chopped

1 tsp fresh ginger, finely chopped

2 stalks celery, chopped

½ small red onion, chopped

1 cup chicken stock (or vegetable if you prefer)

2 tbsp Soy sauce

2 tbsp extra virgin olive oil

Directions:

Cook prawns in a bit of the oil and soy sauce until done and set aside (about 10-15 minutes).

Boil the noodles according the directions (usually 6-8 minutes).

Set aside.

Sauté the vegetables, then add the garlic, ginger, red onion, chilli in a bit of oil until tender and crunchy, but not mushy.

Add the prawns, and noodles, and simmer low about 5-10 minutes past that point.

Chicken with mole salad

Preparation time: 10 minutes | Cooking time: 35 minutes |Servings: 2

Ingredients:

1 skinned chicken breast

2 cups spinach, washed, dried and torn in halves

2 celery stalks, chopped or sliced thinly

½ cup arugula

½ small red onion, diced

2 Medjool pitted dates, chopped

1 tbsp of dark chocolate powder

1 tbsp extra virgin olive oil

2 tbsp Water

5 sprigs of parsley, chopped

Dash of salt

Directions:

In a food processor, blend the dates, chocolate powder, oil and water, and salt.

Add the chilli and process further.

Rub this paste onto the chicken breast, and set it aside, in the refrigerator.

Prepare other salad mixings, the vegetables and herbs in a bowl and toss.

Cook the chicken in a dash of oil in a pan, until done, about 10-15 minutes over a medium burner.

When done, let cool and lay over the salad bed and serve.

Strawberry fields salad

Preparation time: 10 minutes | Cooking time: 20 minutes | Servings: 2

Ingredients:

½ cup cooked buckwheat

1 avocado, pitted, sliced andscooped

1 small tomato, quartered

2 Medjool dates, pitted

5 walnuts, chopped coarsely

20 g red onion

1 tbsp Capers

1 cup arugula

1 cup spinach

3 sprigs parsley, chopped

6 strawberries, sliced

1 tbsp extra virgin olive oil

½ lemon, juiced

1 tbsp Ground turmeric

Directions:

Use room temperature buckwheat or serve warm if preferred.

Wash, dry and chop ingredients above, finish with the lemon and olive oil and turmeric as a dressing.

Add the buckwheat then the strawberries to the top of the salad.

Chilled gazpacho

Preparation time: 10 minutes | Cooking time: 20 minutes | Servings: 2

Ingredients:

2 large, or 6 small tomatoes, chopped

1 avocado, pitted, sliced, and scooped out (wait to do this until instructed)

1 medium cucumber, chopped

1 small red onion, chopped

1 cup of arugula, chopped very finely

½ stalk of celery chopped very finely

1 clove of garlic, minced or pressed

½ chilli or a dash of cayenne pepper

1 tsp lime juice

Dash of sea salt

Dash of pepper

Directions:

Add the ingredients to a blender, or a food processor, and pulse gently.

You do not want to blend too well, or you will make a liquid, as opposed to a soup.

The gazpacho should be chunky.

After blending, put into the refrigerator for about 1 hour.

You can also let this sit overnight.

Just before eating, slice and scoop out the avocado.

Ladle half of the gazpacho into a chilled bowl.

Add the slices of avocado and serve immediately.

Chapter 7: Main dishes

Indian lentil soup

Preparation time: 10 minutes | Cooking time: 50 minutes | Servings: 2

Ingredients:

2 cups of lentils

1 small red onion, minced

1 stalk of celery, finely chopped

1 carrot, chopped

2 large leaves of kale, chopped finely, or 1 cup of baby kale, chopped

2 sprigs of cilantro, minced

3 sprigs of parsley, minced

¼-½ chilli pepper, deseeded and minced (use more or less to your taste)

1 tomato, chopped into small pieces

1 chunk of ginger, minced

1 clove of garlic, minced

5 cups of chicken or vegetable stock

1 tsp of turmeric

1 tsp extra virgin olive oil

½ tsp Salt

Directions:

Cook lentils according to the package, removing from heat about 5 minutes before they would be done.

In a saucepan, sauté all of the vegetables in the olive oil.

Then add the chopped greens last.

Then add the ginger, garlic, and chilli and turmeric powder.

Add the stock and simmer for 5 minutes.

Add the lentils, and salt.

Stir in the precooked lentils and cook longer, on a very low simmer, for 25 more minutes.

Remove from the heat and cool.

Cut the avocado, remove the pit, and slice it, then scoop out the slices just before eating.

Top with avocado slice, then serve immediately.

Shrimp & arugula soup

Preparation time: 5 minutes | Cooking time: 30 minutes | Servings: 3

Ingredients:

10 medium sized shrimp or 5 large prawns, cleaned, deshelled and deveined

1 small red onion, sliced very thinly

1 cup arugula

1 cup baby kale

2 large celery stalks, sliced very thinly

5 sprigs of parsley, chopped

11 cloves of garlic, minced

5 cups of chicken or fish or vegetable stock

1 tbsp extra virgin olive oil

Dash of sea salt

Dash of pepper

Directions:

Sauté the vegetables (not the kale or arugula just yet however), in a stock pot, on low heat for about 2 minutes so that they are still tender and still crunchy, but not cooked quite yet.

You will need to save the cooking time for the next step.

Add the salt and pepper.

Next, clean and chop the shrimp into bite-sized pieces that would be comfortable eating in a soup.

Then, add the shrimp to the pot, and sauté for 10 more minutes on medium-low heat.

Make sure the shrimp is cooked thoroughly and is not translucent.

When the shrimp seems to be cooked through, add the stock to the pot and cook on medium for about 20 more minutes.

Remove from heat and cool before serving.

Creamy chicken soup

Preparation time: 5 minutes | Cooking time: 30 minutes | Servings: 3

Ingredients:

4 chicken breasts

1 carrot, chopped

1 cup zucchini, peeled and chopped

2 cups cauliflower, broken into florets

1 celery rib, chopped

1 small onion, chopped

5 cups water

½ tsp salt

Black pepper, to taste

Directions:

Place chicken breasts, onion, carrot, celery, cauliflower and zucchini in a deep soup pot.

Add in salt, black pepper and 5 cups of water.

Stir and bring to a boil.

Simmer for 30 minutes then remove chicken from the pot and let it cool slightly.

Blend soup until completely smooth.

Shred or dice the chicken meat, return it back to the pot, stir, and serve.

Broccoli and chicken soup

Preparation time: 5 minutes | Cooking time: 30 minutes | Servings: 3

Ingredients:

4 boneless chicken thighs, diced

1 small carrot, chopped

1 broccoli head, broken into florets

1 garlic clove, chopped

1 small onion, chopped

4 cups water

3 tbsp extra virgin olive oil

½ tsp salt

Black pepper, to taste

Directions:

In a deep soup pot, heat olive oil and gently sauté broccoli for 2-3 minutes, stirring occasionally.

Add in onion, carrot, chicken and cook, stirring, for 2-3 minutes. Stir in salt, black pepper and water.

Bring to a boil. Simmer for 30 minutes then remove from heat and set aside to cool.

In a blender or food processor, blend soup until completely smooth. Serve and enjoy!

Warm chicken and avocado soup

Preparation time: 5 minutes | Cooking time: 30 minutes | Servings: 3

Ingredients:

2 ripe avocados, peeled and chopped

1 cooked chicken breast, shredded

1 garlic clove, chopped

3 cups chicken broth

Salt and black pepper, to taste

Fresh coriander leaves, finely cut, to serve

½ cup sour cream, to serve

Directions:

Combine avocados, garlic, and chicken broth in a blender.

Process until smooth and transfer to a saucepan.

Add in chicken and cook, stirring, over medium heat until the mixture is hot.

Serve topped with sour cream and finely cut coriander leaves.

Healthy chicken and oat soup

Preparation time: 5 minutes | Cooking time: 40 minutes | Servings: 3

Ingredients:

3 chicken breasts, diced

1 small onion, chopped

3 garlic cloves

½ cup quick-cooking oats

1 large carrot, chopped

1 red bell pepper, chopped

1 celery rib, chopped

1 tomato, diced

5 cups water

1 bay leaf

1 tsp salt

½ cup fresh parsley leaves, finely cut

Black pepper, to taste

Directions:

Place the chicken, bay leaf, celery, carrot, onion, red pepper, tomato and salt into a soup pot.

Add in water and bring to the boil then reduce heat and simmer for 30 minutes.

Discard the bay leaf, season with salt and pepper, add in the oats and parsley, simmer for 5 more minutes, and serve.

Asparagus and chicken soup

Preparation time: 5 minutes | Cooking time: 30 minutes | Servings: 3

Ingredients:

2 chicken breast fillets, cooked and diced

2-3 leeks, finely cut

1 bunch asparagus, trimmed and cut

4 cups chicken broth

2 tbsp extra virgin olive oil

½ cup fresh parsley, finely chopped

Salt and black pepper, to taste

Lemon juice, to serve

Directions:

Heat the olive oil in a large soup pot.

Add in the leeks and gently sauté, stirring, for 2-3 minutes.

Add chicken broth, the diced chicken, and bring to a boil.

Reduce heat and simmer for 15 minutes.

Add in asparagus, parsley, salt and black pepper, and cook for 5 minutes more.

Serve with lemon juice.

Mediterranean fish and quinoa soup

Preparation time: 5 minutes | Cooking time: 40 minutes | Servings: 3

Ingredients:

1Lb cod fillets, cubed

1 onion, chopped

3 tomatoes, chopped

½ cup quinoa, rinsed

1 red pepper, chopped

1 carrot, chopped

½ cup black olives, pitted and sliced

1 garlic clove, crushed

3 tbsp extra virgin olive oil

A pinch of cayenne pepper

1 bay leaf

1 tsp dried thyme

1 tsp dried dill

½ tsp pepper

½ cup white wine

4 cups water

Salt and black pepper, totaste

½ cup fresh parsley, finelycut

Directions:

Heat the olive oil over medium heat and sauté the onion, red pepper, garlic and carrot until tender.

Stir in the cayenne pepper, bay leaf, herbs, salt and pepper.

Add the white wine, water, quinoa and tomatoes and bring to a boil.

Reduce heat, cover, and cook for 10 minutes.

Stir in olives and the fish and cook for another 10 minutes.

Stir in parsley and serve hot.

Bean stew

Preparation time: 5 minutes | Cooking time: 35 minutes | Servings: 3

Ingredients:

50g of kale, chopped roughly

½ bird's eye chilli, chopped finely (optional)

40g of buckwheat

50g of red onion, chopped finely

1 garlic clove, chopped finely

1 tbsp of roughly chopped parsley

200ml vegetable stock

1 tsp of herbes de provence

200g of tinned mixed beans

1 tsp of tomato purée

1 x 400g tin of chopped Italian tomatoes

30g celery, trimmed and chopped finely

1 tbsp of extra virgin olive oil

30g of carrot, peeled and chopped finely

Directions:

Heat the oil in a medium sized saucepan placed over medium low heat.

Add in the onion, celery, chilli, carrot, garlic and herbs (if using) until the onions are soft enough but not coloured.

Add the stock, tomato purée, and tomatoes and bring to a boil.

Put in the beans and allow for 30 minutes simmering.

Add the kales and cook for 5-10 minutes or until the kale is tender, and then add in parsley. As it cools, cook the buckwheat as per the directions on the packet.

Drain the buckwheat and serve with the cooked stew.

Pork with pak choi

Preparation time: 5 minutes | Cooking time: 40 minutes | Servings: 3

Ingredients:

100g of shiitake mushrooms, sliced

1 tbsp of corn flour

200g pak choi or choi sum-cut into thin slices

125ml of chicken stock

1 tbsp of tomato purée

1 tsp of brown sugar

1 clove garlic, peeled and crushed

1 shallot, peeled and sliced

100g of bean sprouts

1 tbsp of water

400g of pork mince (10% fat)

1 thumb (5cm) fresh ginger -peeled and grated

400g of firm tofu, cut into large cubes

1 tbsp of rice wine

1 tbsp of soy sauce

A large handful (20g) of parsley, chopped

1 tbsp of rapeseed oil

Directions:

Place the tofu on kitchen paper, cover it with kitchen paper, and then set it aside.

In a small bowl, mix water and corn flour and remove the lumps.

Add in rice wine, brown sugar, chicken stock, tomato puree, and soy sauce.

Also, add in the crushed ginger and garlic them mix.

Place a large frying pan or wok on high heat and add oil to it.

Add the mushrooms and stir-fry for 2 to 3 minutes until cooked and glossy.

Using a slotted spoon, remove the mushrooms from the pan and let them rest.

Add tofu to the pan, fry it until it is brown on all sides, remove it with a slotted spoon when done and set aside.

Add the pak choi to your pan or wok, and stir-fry for about 2 minutes and, then add the mince.

Cook it until it cooks through and then add the sauce.

Reduce the heat a notch and allow the sauce to bubble around the meat for 1-2 minutes.

Add the tofu, beansprouts, and mushrooms to the pan and warm them all through.

Remove it from the heat and mix in parsley then serve right away.

Chicken soup

Preparation time: 5 minutes | Cooking time: 30 minutes | Servings: 3

Ingredients:

1 tsp of smoked paprika

300ml passata

Salt and freshly ground black pepper

1 tsp of dried mixed herbs

1 x 400g can of black beans, drained

2 cloves garlic, peeled and crushed

1 carrot, peeled and roughly chopped

1 litre of water

1 tsp of mild chilli powder

1 red chilli, deseeded then finely chopped

½ tsp of turmeric

30g (large handful) of flat leaf parsley, chopped

1 x 400g can chopped tomatoes

1 tsp of paprika

½ tsp of ground cumin

1 green pepper, deseeded and chopped

1 x 400g can kidney beans, drained

4 chicken drumsticks

2 shallots, peeled then roughly chopped

Directions:

Take a large saucepan and add in the chicken drumsticks, carrot, and shallots.

Pour in the water and let it simmer.

Allow to cook for 20 minutes, and then remove the chicken drumsticks with a spoon (slotted) and set it aside to cool.

Add in the chopped tomatoes, garlic, passata, chilli, and green pepper, and let it simmer again.

Put in the dried herbs, paprika, turmeric, smoked paprika, chilli powder, and cumin, then simmer again for 30 minutes.

Pull off the skin from the chicken then pinch as much chicken as possible from the bone.

Shred the chicken meat, place it on the pan along with the kidney beans and black beans, and cook for five minutes.

Remove from the heat, add parsley, and stir it in.

Season with pepper and salt (to taste).

Beef with red wine and herb-roasted potatoes

Preparation time: 5 minutes | Cooking time: 60 minutes | Servings: 3

Ingredients:

40ml of red wine

1 tbsp of extra virgin olive oil

1 clove of garlic, finely chopped

5g of parsley, finely chopped

50g of red onions-sliced to rings

50g of sliced kale

1 tsp of corn flour dissolved in 1 tbsp of water

100g of potatoes, peeled then cut into 2cm chunks

150Ml of beef stock

1 tsp of tomato purée

150G of beefsteak

Directions:

Preheat your oven to 220 degrees.

Boil the potatoes for 5 minutes then drain.

Place them in a roasting tin together with a tsp of oil and let them roast for 35 to 45 minutes.

Make sure to turn them every ten minutes.

Once done, take them out and mix them with parsley.

Over medium heat, fry the onion in a tsp of oil for 5 to 7 minutes.

Steam the kale for 2 to 3 minutes then drain.

Fry the garlic in a tsp of oil for a minute, add the kale, and stir-fry for 1 to 2 more minutes.

Smear the beef with ½ tsp of oil and fry it in a hot pan over medium heat until cooked as desired.

Remove it and set aside.

Pour wine onto the hot pan and reduce the heat to simmer the wine until syrupy.

Add tomato purée and stock, let it boil, and add the corn flour paste to thicken.

Serve the beef with onion rings, roast potatoes, red wine sauce, kale, and enjoy.

Salmon salad with mint dressing

Preparation time: 5 minutes | Cooking time: 30 minutes | Servings: 3

Ingredients:

1 small handful (10g) of parsley, chopped roughly

2 radishes, trimmed and thinlysliced

40g of young spinach leaves

5cm piece (50g) cucumber, cut into chunks

40g of mixed salad leaves

2 spring onions, trimmed then sliced

1 salmon fillet (130g)

For the dressing:

1 tbsp of rice vinegar

1 tsp of low-fat mayonnaise

Salt and freshly ground black pepper, to taste 2MInt leaves, finely chopped

1 tbsp of natural yoghurt

Directions:

Preheat your oven to 200 degrees. Place salmon fillets on a baking tray and allow them to bake for about 16-18 minutes.

Remove from the oven and then let them rest (salmon is ok served hot or cold when added to the salad).

Remove the skin of your salmon (if it has one) after cooking.

Mix the mayonnaise, mint leaves, rice wine vinegar, salt, yoghurt, and pepper in a small bowl and let it stand for 5 minutes to let the flavour deepen.

Place the salad leaves with the spinach on top of a plate and top with the radishes, spring onions, cucumber, and parsley.

Flake the salmon onto the salad then drizzle the dressing over.

Hearty quinoa and spinach breakfast casserole

Preparation time: 5 minutes | Cooking time: 20 minutes | Servings: 3

Ingredients:

1 cup cooked quinoa

3-4 spring onions, finely chopped

5 oz frozen chopped spinach, thawed and squeezed dry

½ zucchini, peeled and shredded

5 eggs

½ cup milk

4 tbsp extra virgin olive oil

salt and black pepper, to taste

1 cup cheddar cheese, grated

Directions:

In a large bowl combine eggs, milk, salt and pepper.

In a deep casserole dish heat the olive oil.

Cook the onions, zucchini and spinach, stirring constantly, until lightly cooked.

Add in the quinoa and combine everything well.

Pour the egg mixture over and then top with cheddar cheese.

Bake in a preheated to 350 f oven for 20 minutes.

Quick quinoa vegetable scramble

Preparation time: 5 minutes | Cooking time: 30 minutes | Servings: 3

Ingredients:

½ cup cooked quinoa

½ small onion, chopped

2 tomatoes, diced

1 large red pepper, chopped

5 eggs

½ cup crumbled feta

4 tbsp extra virgin olive oil

Black pepper, to taste

Salt, to taste

Directions:

In a large pan, sauté onion over medium heat for 1-2 minutes, stirring.

Add in tomatoes and red pepper and cook until the mixture is almost dry.

Stir in quinoa, feta and eggs and cook until well mixed and not too liquid.

Season with black pepper and serve.

Coconut and quinoa banana pudding

Preparation time: 5 minutes | Cooking time: 30 minutes | Servings: 3

Ingredients:

1 cup quinoa

3 cups coconut milk

3 ripe bananas

¼ cup flaked unsweetened coconut

4 tbsp sugar

1 tsp vanilla extract

Directions:

Wash and cook quinoa according to package directions.

When ready remove from heat and set aside.

In a separate bowl blend sugar, milk and bananas until smooth.

Add to the quinoa.

Heat over medium heat, string, until creamy.

Stir in vanilla and coconut flakes and serve warm.

Chicken with kale and chilli salsa

Preparation time: 5 minutes | Cooking time: 40 minutes| Servings: 3

Ingredients: 50g of buckwheat

1 tsp of chopped fresh ginger

Juice of ½ lemon, divided

2 tsp of ground turmeric

50g of kale, chopped 20g red onion, sliced

120g of skinless, boneless chicken breast

1 tbsp of extra virgin olive oil

1 tomato 1 handful parsley

1 bird's eye chilli, chopped

Directions: Start with the salsa: remove the eye out of the tomato and finely chop it, making sure to keep as much of the liquid as you can. Mix it with the chilli, parsley, and lemon juice.

You could add everything to a blender for different results.

Heat your oven to 220F.

Marinate the chicken with a little oil, 1 tsp of turmeric, and the lemon juice.

Let it rest for 5-10 minutes.

Heat a pan over medium heat until it is hot then add marinated chicken and allow it to cook for a minute on both sides until it is pale gold).

Transfer the chicken to the oven (if pan is not ovenproof place it in a baking tray) and bake for 8 to 10 minutes or until it is cooked through.

Take the chicken out of the oven, cover with foil, and let it rest for five minutes before you serve.

Meanwhile, in a steamer, steam the kale for about 5 minutes.

In a little oil, fry the ginger and red onions until they are soft but not coloured, and then add in the cooked kale and fry it for a minute.

Cook the buckwheat in accordance to the packet directions with the remaining turmeric.

Serve alongside the vegetables, salsa and chicken.

Sirt salmon salad

Preparation time: 5 minutes | Cooking time: 30 minutes | Servings: 3

Ingredients:

1 large Medjool date, pitted then chopped

50g of chicory leaves

50g of rocket

1 tbsp of extra virgin olive oil

10g of parsley, chopped

10g of celery leaves, chopped

40g of celery, sliced

15G of walnuts, chopped

1 tbsp of capers

20g of red onions-sliced

80g of avocado-peeled, stoned, and sliced

Juice of ¼ lemon

100g of smoked salmon slices (alternatives: lentils, tinned tuna, or cooked chicken breast)

Directions:

Arrange all the salad leaves on a large plate then mix the rest of the ingredients and distribute evenly on top the leaves.

Greek salad skewers

Preparation time: 5 minutes | Cooking time: 30 minutes | Servings: 3

Ingredients:

100g of cucumber, cut into 4 slices and halved (about 10cm)

8 cherry tomatoes

100g feta, cut into 8 cubes

8 large black olives

1 yellow pepper, cut into 8 squares

½ red onion, cut in half and separated into 8 pieces

2 wooden skewers, soaked in water for 30 minutes before use

For the dressing:

Juice of ½ lemon

½ garlic clove, peeled and crushed

1 tbsp of extra virgin olive oil

A few leaves of finely chopped basil

Generous seasoning of salt and freshly ground black pepper a few finely chopped oregano leaves

1 tsp of balsamic vinegar

Directions:

Thread every skewer with salad ingredients in this order; olive, followed by tomato, then yellow pepper, red onion, followed by cucumber then feta, tomato, olive, then yellow pepper, red onion and finally cucumber.

Place the dressing ingredients in a small bowl, mix them thoroughly, and then pour over the skewers.

Alkalizing green soup

Preparation time: 5 minutes | Cooking time: 40 minutes | Servings: 3

Ingredients:

2 cups broccoli, cut into florets and chopped

2 zucchinis, peeled and chopped

2 cups chopped kale

1 small onion, chopped

2-3 garlic cloves, chopped

4 cups vegetable broth

2 tbsp extra virgin olive oil

½ tsp ground ginger

½ tsp ground coriander

1 lime, juiced, to serve

Directions:

Gently heat olive oil in a large saucepan over medium-high heat.

Cook onion and garlic for 3-4 minutes until tender.

Add ginger and coriander and stir to coat well.

Add in broccoli, zucchinis, kale and vegetable broth.

Bring to the boil, then reduce heat and simmer for 15 minutes, stirring from time to time.

Set aside to cool and blend until smooth.

Return to pan and cook until heated through. Serve with lime juice.

1 cup raw cashews

1 cup vegetable broth

4 cups water

3 tbsp extra virgin olive oil

½ tsp ground nutmeg

Directions:

Soak cashews in a bowl covered with water for at least 4 hours.

Drain water and blend cashews with 1 cup of vegetable broth until smooth.

Set aside.

Gently heat olive oil in a large saucepan over medium-high heat.

Cook onion and garlic for 3-4 minutes until tender.

Add in broccoli, potato, nutmeg and water.

Cover and bring to the boil, then reduce heat and simmer for 20 minutes, stirring from time to time.

Remove from heat and stir in cashew mixture.

Blend until smooth, return to pan andcook until heated through.

Creamy broccoli and potato soup

Preparation time: 5 minutes | Cooking time: 30 minutes | Servings: 3

Ingredients:

3 cups broccoli, cut into florets and chopped

2 potatoes, peeled and chopped

1 large onion, chopped

3 garlic cloves, minced

Creamy brussels sprout soup

Preparation time: 5 minutes | Cooking time: 35 minutes | Servings: 3

Ingredients:

1Lb frozen brussels sprouts, thawed

2 potatoes, peeled and chopped

1 large onion, chopped

3 garlic cloves, minced

1 cup raw cashews

4 cups vegetable broth

3 tbsp extra virgin olive oil

½ tsp curry powder

Salt and black pepper, to taste

Directions:

Soak cashews in a bowl covered with water for at least 4 hours.

Drain water and blend cashews with 1 cup of vegetable broth until smooth.

Set aside.

Gently heat olive oil in a large saucepan over medium-high heat.

Cook onion and garlic and for 3-4 minutes until tender.

Add in brussels sprouts, potato, curry and vegetable broth.

Cover and bring to a boil, then reduce heat and simmer for 20 minutes, stirring from time to time.

Remove from heat and stir in cashew mixture.

Blend until smooth, return to pan andcook until heated through.

Chicken and arugula salad with Italian dressing

Preparation time: 5 minutes | Cooking time: 30 minutes | Servings: 3

Ingredients:

6oz. of chicken (or turkey), skinless, boneless grilled or prepared in theskillet

Large mixed arugula and lettuce salad

½ cup Italian dressing

½ tsp of mustard

Tuna with arugula salad with Italian dressing

6 oz. Can of tuna, drained.

Large mixed arugula

Red onion salad

½ cup italian dressing

½ tsp of mustard

You may use fish sauce instead of salt

Avocado and chicken risotto

Preparation time: 5 minutes | Cooking time: 20 minutes | Servings: 3

Ingredients:

3 cups chicken broth

2 chicken breasts, diced

1 cup risotto rice

2 avocados, peeled and diced

3 tbsp extra virgin olive oil

1 onion, finely chopped

2 garlic cloves, crushed

2 tbsp raisins

1 cup grated parmesan cheese, plus extra to serve

5-6 green onions, finely cut, to serve

Directions:

Place chicken broth in a saucepan, bring to the boil, then reduce heat to low and keep at a simmer.

In a non-stick fry pan, cook chicken for 5-6 minutes each side, or until browned and cooked through.

Transfer to a plate in the same pan, heat olive oil over medium heat.

Add the onion and cook, stirring, for 1-2 minutes until softened.

Stir in the garlic, then add the rice and cook, stirring, for 1 minute to coat the grains.

Add the broth, a spoonful at a time, stirring occasionally, allowing each spoonful to be absorbed before adding the next.

Simmer until all liquid has absorbed and rice is tender.

Stir in the chicken, parmesan cheese and raisins, then cover and remove from the heat.

Serve in bowls topped with diced avocados, extra parmesan cheese and chopped green onions.

Chicken and chickpea fritters

Preparation time: 5 minutes | Cooking time: 30 minutes | Servings: 3

Ingredients:

1 can chickpeas, drained

2 chicken breasts, cooked and shredded

2 egg whites

½ cup fresh parsley leaves, very finely cut

1 tsp ginger

½ tsp black pepper salt, to taste

2 tbsp coconut oil, for frying

Directions:

Blend the chickpeas in a food processor and combine them with the chicken, egg whites, parsley, and ginger into a smooth batter.

Heat the oil in a frying pan over medium heat.

Using a large tbsp, form the batter into fritters.

Cook each one for 2-3 minutes each side or until golden and cooked through.

Chicken and lentil stew

Preparation time: 5 minutes | Cooking time: 50 minutes | Servings: 3

Ingredients:

4 chicken breasts, diced

½ cup red lentils, rinsed

1 carrot, chopped 1 small onion, chopped

1 garlic clove, chopped

1 celery stalk, chopped

1 small red pepper, chopped

1 can tomatoes, chopped 1 tbsp paprika

1 tsp ginger, grated

3 tbsp extra virgin olive oil

½ cup fresh parsley leaves, finely cut, to serve

Directions:

Heat olive oil in a casserole and gently brown the chicken, stirring.

Add in onions, garlic, celery, carrot, pepper, paprika and ginger.

Cook, stirring constantly, for 2-3 minutes.

Add in the lentils and tomatoes and bring to a boil.

Lower heat, cover, and simmer for 30 minutes, or until the lentils are tender and the chicken is cooked through.

Serve sprinkled with fresh parsley.

Brussels sprouts egg skillet

Preparation time: 5 minutes | Cooking time: 30 minutes | Servings: 3

Ingredients:

½lb brussels sprouts, halved

1 small onion, chopped

10 cherry tomatoes, halved

4 eggs

1 tbsp extra virgin olive oil

Directions:

In an 8 inch cast iron skillet, heat olive oil over medium heat.

Add in onion and sauté for 1-2 minutes.

Add in brussels sprouts and tomatoes and season with salt and pepper to taste.

Cook for 3-4 minutes then crack the eggs, cover and cook until egg whites have set, and egg yolk is desired consistency.

Salmon kebabs

Preparation time: 5 minutes | Cooking time: 20 minutes | Servings: 3

Ingredients:

2 shallots, ends trimmed, halved

2 zucchinis, cut in 2-inch cubes

1 cup cherry tomatoes

6 skinless salmon fillets, cut into 1-inch pieces

3 limes, cut into thin wedges

Directions:

Preheat barbecue or char grill on medium-high.

Thread fish cubes onto skewers, then zucchinis, shallots and tomatoes.

Repeat to make 12 kebabs.

Bake the kebabs for about 3 minutes each side for medium cooked.

Transfer to a plate, cover with foil and set aside for 5 min to rest.

Mediterranean baked salmon

Preparation time: 5 minutes | Cooking time: 30 minutes | Servings: 3

Ingredients:

2 (6 oz) boneless salmon fillets

1 tomato, thinly sliced

1 onion, thinly sliced

1 tbsp capers

3 tbsp olive oil

1 tsp dry oregano

3 tbsp parmesan cheese

Salt and black pepper, to taste

Directions:

Preheat oven to 350F.

Place the salmon fillets in a baking dish, sprinkle with oregano, top with onion and tomato slices, drizzle with olive oil, and sprinkle with capers and parmesan cheese.

Cover the dish with foil and bake for 30 minutes, or until the fish flakes easily.

Simple oven-baked sea bass

Preparation time: 5 minutes | Cooking time: 50 minutes | Servings: 3

Ingredients:

1Lb sea bass, cleaned and scaled

5 oz fennel, trimmed and sliced

5-6 spring onions, chopped

2 garlic cloves, chopped

10 black olives, pitted and halved

2-3 lemon wedges

1 tbsp capers

2 garlic cloves, finely chopped

½ tsp paprika

½ cup dry white wine

3 tbsp extra virgin olive oil

Salt and pepper, to taste

Directions:

In a cup, mix garlic, olive oil, salt, and black pepper.

Arrange the sliced fennel in a shallow ovenproof casserole.

Add the green onions and lay the fish on top.

Pour over the olive mixture.

Scatter the olives, paprika and lemon wedges over the fish, then pour the wine over.

Cover the dish with a lid or foil and bake for 20 minutes, or until the fish flakes easily.

Lemon rosemary fish fillets

Preparation time: 5 minutes | Cooking time: 30 minutes | Servings: 3

Ingredients:

4 white fish fillets

1 tbsp dried rosemary

4 tbsp breadcrumbs

2 tbsp lemon zest

1 tsp garlic powder

2 tbsp extra virgin olive oil

1 tsp salt

Directions:

Combine the rosemary, breadcrumbs, lemon zest, garlic powder and salt in a food processor and blend until well mixed.

Place the fish fillets, skin-side up, on a lined baking tray.

Grill for 3-4 minutes.

Turn the fish over and press a quarter of the breadcrumb mixture over the top of each fillet.

Drizzle with olive oil and grill for 4 min until the crust is golden and the fish is cooked through.

Serve with steamed spinach or baked potatoes.

Asian salmon with broccoli

Preparation time: 5 minutes | Cooking time: 40 minutes | Servings: 3

Ingredients:

4 salmon fillets, skin on

1 lb fresh broccoli florets

2 tbsp soy sauce

2 tbsp toasted sesame oil

1 tsp chilli garlic sauce

1 tbsp brown sugar

½ cup green onions, finely cut, to serve

Directions:

In a large bowl, combine the garlic and soy sauce with the sesame oil and brown sugar.

Add in the salmon and broccoli and toss to coat.

Place salmon skin side down in a single layer on a lined baking tray.

Add the broccoli florets around.

Bake 10-12 minutes or until the fish is cooked through and flakes easily with a fork.

Top with green onions and serve.

Salmon and spinach with feta cheese

Preparation time: 5 minutes | Cooking time: 30 minutes | Servings: 3

Ingredients:

4 salmon fillets, skin on

1 bag frozen spinach

4-5 green onions, chopped

1 cup crumbled feta cheese

4 tbsp extra virgin olive oil

Salt and pepper, to taste

Lemon wedges, to serve

Directions:

In a skillet, heat olive oil on medium-high.

Cook the spinach and the green onions for 2-3 min, stirring once or twice.

Season with salt and pepper to taste and add in the feta cheese.

Cook for 1 minute more.

Place salmon skin side down in a single layer on a lined baking tray and roast for 10-12 minutes or until it is cooked through and flakes easily with a fork.

Spoon the spinach mixture onto plates, then top with the salmon and serve with lemon wedges.

Chapter 8: Snacks and juices

Sirt fruit salad

Preparation time: 5 minutes | Cooking time: 0 minutes |Servings: 3

Ingredients:

½ cup crisply made green tea

1 tsp nectar

1 orange, divided

1 apple, cored and generally slashed

10 red seedless grapes

10 blueberries

Directions:

Stir the nectar into a large portion of some green tea.

When broken down, include the juice of a large portion of the orange.

Leave to cool.

Chop the other portion of the orange and spot in a bowl together with the cleaved apple, grapes and blueberries.

Pour over the cooled tea and leave to soak for a couple of moments before serving.

Raspberry and blackcurrant jelly

Preparation time: 5 minutes | Cooking time: 0 minutes | Servings: 3

Ingredients:

100g raspberries, washed

2 leaves gelatine

100g blackcurrants, washed and stalks evacuated

2 tbsp granulated sugar

300ml water

Directions:

Arrange the raspberries in two serving dishes/glasses/moulds.

Put the gelatine leaves in a bowl of cold water to soften.

Place the blackcurrants in a little container with the sugar and 100ml water and bring to the bubble.

Stew vivaciously for 5 minutes and afterward expel from the warmth.

Leave to represent 2 minutes.

Squeeze out overabundance water from the gelatine leaves and add them to the pot.

Mix until completely broke up, then mix in the remainder of the water.

Empty the fluid into the readied dishes and refrigerate to set.

The jams ought to be prepared in around 3-4 hours or medium-term.

Apple pancakes with blackcurrant compote

Preparation time: 5 minutes | Cooking time: 20 minutes | Servings: 3

Ingredients:

75g porridge oats sirtfood plans

125g plain flour

1 tsp heating powder

2 tbsp caster sugar

Spot of salt

2 apples, stripped, cored and cut into little pieces

300ml semi-skimmed milk

2 egg whites

2 tsp light olive oil

For the compote:

120g blackcurrants, washed and stalks expelled

2 tbsp caster sugar

3 tbsp water

Directions:

First make the compote.

Spot the blackcurrants, sugar and water in a little dish.

Raise to a stew and cook for 10-15 minutes.

Place the oats, flour, heating powder, caster sugar and salt in a huge bowl and blend well.

Mix in the apple and afterward rush in the milk a little at once until you have a smooth blend.

Whisk the egg whites to stiff pinnacles and afterward crease into the hotcake player.

Move the player to a container.

Heat ½ tsp oil in a non-stick skillet on a medium-high warmth and pour in around one fourth of the hitter.

Cook on the two sides until brilliant dark coloured. Evacuate and rehash to make four hotcakes.

Serve the flapjacks with the blackcurrant compote sprinkled over

Quinoa and date cookies

Preparation time: 5 minutes | Cooking time: 30 minutes | Servings: 3

Ingredients:

½ cup almond flour

½ cup cooked quinoa

1/3 cup brown sugar

½ cup butter

4 tbsp tahini

16 dates, pitted and chopped

1 tsp baking soda

½ tsp vanilla extract

Directions:

Preheat oven to 350F.

Combine sugar, tahini and butter stirring until creamy.

Add in remaining

Ingredients. Mix very well.

Spoon rounded teaspoonfuls of dough onto cookie sheets.

Bake for 10-12 minutes, or until cookies start to turn golden brown.

The sirtfood diet green juice

Preparation time: 5 minutes | Cooking time: 0 minutes | Servings: 3

Ingredients:

(2 enormous bunches) kale

30 g (an enormous bunch) rocket

5 g (a little bunch) level leaf parsley

5 g (a little bunch) lovage leaves (discretionary)

Enormous stalks green celery, including leaves

A large portion of a medium green apple

A large portion of a lemon, squeezed

Matcha green tea

Directions:

Blend the greens (kale, rocket, parsley, and lovage, on the off chance that utilizing) together, at that point juice them.

We discover juicers can truly vary in their proficiency at squeezing verdant vegetables and you may need to re-squeeze the leftovers before proceeding onward to different fixings.

The objective is to wind up with about 50ml of juice from the greens.

Presently squeeze the celery and the apple

You can strip the lemon and put it through the juicer also, however, we think that it's a lot simpler to just press the lemon by hand into the juice.

By this stage, you ought to have around 250ML of juice altogether, maybe somewhat more.

It is just when the juice is made and prepared to serve that you include the matcha green tea.

Pour a modest quantity of the juice into a glass, at that point include the matcha and mix vivaciously with a fork or tsp.

We just use matcha in the initial two beverages of the day as it contains moderate measures of caffeine (a similar substance as a typical cup of tea).

For individuals not accustomed to it, it might keep them alert whenever alcoholic late.

Once the match is broken down include the rest of the juice.

Give it a last mix, at that point, your juice is prepared to drink.

Don't hesitate to top up with plain water, as indicated by taste.

Kale and blackcurrant smoothie

Preparation time: 5 minutes | Cooking time: 0 minutes | Servings: 3

Ingredients: 2 tsp nectar

1 cup crisply made green tea

10 infant kale leaves, stalks evacuated

1 ready banana

40 g blackcurrants, washed and stalks evacuated

6 ice solid shapes

Directions:

Mix the nectar into the warm green tea until broke down.

Wonder every one of the fixings together in a blender until smooth.

Serve right away.

Green tea smoothie

Preparation time: 5 minutes | Cooking time: 0 minutes | Servings: 3

Ingredients:

2 ready bananas

250 ml milk

2 tsp matcha green tea powder

½ tsp vanilla bean glue (not separate) or a little scratch of the seeds from a vanilla unit

6 ice 3D squares

2 tsp nectar

Directions:

Mix every one of the fixings together in a blender and serve in two glasses.

Raw vegan fruits dipped in superfoods chocolate

Preparation time: 5 minutes | Cooking time: 0 minutes | Servings: 3

Ingredients:

2 apples or 2 bananas or a bowl of strawberries or any fruit that can be dipped in melted chocolate

½ cup of melted superfoods chocolate (see earlier recipe)

2 tbsp chopped nuts (almond, walnut, brazil nuts) or seeds (hemp, chia, sesame, flax meal)

Directions:

Cut apple in wedges or cut banana in quarters.

Melt the chocolate and chop the nuts.

Dip fruit in chocolate, sprinkle with nuts or seeds and lay on tray.

Transfer the tray to the fridge so the chocolate can harden; serve.

If you don't want chocolate, cover fruits with almond or sunflower butter and sprinkle with chia or hemp seeds, cut it into chunks and serve.

Fruit skewers & strawberry dip

Preparation time: 5 minutes| Cooking time: 0 minutes| Servings: 3

Ingredients:

150G (5oz) red grapes

1 pineapple, (approx. 2Lb weight) peeled and diced

400g (14oz) strawberries

Directions:

Place 100g (3½ oz) of the strawberries into a food processor and blend until smooth.

Pour the dip into a serving bowl.

Skewer the grapes, pineapple chunks and remaining strawberries onto skewers.

Serve alongside the strawberry dip.

Choc nut truffles

Preparation time: 5 minutes | Cooking time: 0 minutes | Servings: 3

Ingredients:

150G (5oz) desiccated (shredded) coconut

50g (2oz) walnuts, chopped

25G (1OZ) hazelnuts, chopped

4 Medjool dates

2 tbsp 100% cocoa powder or cacao nibs

1 tbsp coconut oil

Directions:

Place all of the ingredients into a blender and process until smooth and creamy.

Using a tsp, scoop the mixture into bite-size pieces then roll it into balls.

Place them into small paper cases, cover them and chill for 1 hour before serving.

No-bake strawberry flapjacks

Preparation time: 5 minutes | Cooking time: 30 minutes | Servings: 3

Ingredients:

75g (3oz) porridge oats

125g (4oz) dates

50g (2oz) strawberries

50g (2oz) peanuts (unsalted)

50g (2oz) walnuts

1 tbsp coconut oil

2 tbsp 100% cocoa powder or cacao nibs

Directions:

Place all of the ingredients into a blender and process until they become a soft consistency.

Spread the mixture onto a baking sheet or small flat tin.

Press the mixture down and smooth it out.

Cut it into 8 pieces, ready to serve.

You can add an extra sprinkling of cocoa powder to garnish if you wish.

Chocolate balls

Preparation time: 5 minutes | Cooking time: 10 minutes | Servings: 3

Ingredients:

50g (2OZ) peanut butter (or almond butter)

25G (1OZ) cocoa powder

25G (1OZ) desiccated (shredded) coconut

1 tbsp honey

1 tbsp cocoa powder for coating

Directions:

Place the ingredients into a bowl and mix.

Using a tsp scoop out a little of the mixture and shape it into a ball.

Roll the ball in a little cocoa powder and set aside.

Repeat for the remaining mixture.

Can be eaten straight away or stored in the fridge.

Warm berries & cream

Preparation time: 5 minutes | Cooking time: 0 minutes | Servings: 3

Ingredients

250G (9oz) blueberries

250G (9oz) strawberries

100g (3½ oz) redcurrants

100g (3½ oz) blackberries

4 tbsp fresh whipped cream

1 tbsp honey

Zest and juice of

1 orange

Directions

Place all of the berries into a pan along with the honey and orange juice.

Gently heat the berries for around 5 minutes until warmed through.

Serve the berries into bowls and add a dollop of whipped cream on top.

Alternatively, you could top them off with fromage frais or yoghurt.

Chocolate fondue

Preparation time: 5 minutes | Cooking time: 10 minutes | Servings: 3

Ingredients:

125g (4oz) dark chocolate (min 85% cocoa)

300g (11oz) strawberries

200g (7oz) cherries

2 apples, peeled, cored and sliced

100ml (3½ fl oz) double cream (heavy cream)

Directions:

Place the chocolate and cream into a fonduc pot or saucepan and warm it until smooth and creamy.

Serve in the fondue pot or transfer it to a serving bowl.

Scatter the fruit on a serving dish ready to be dipped into the chocolate.

Walnut & date loaf

Preparation time: 5 minutes | Cooking time: 30 minutes | Servings: 3

Ingredients:

250G (9oz) self-rising flour

125g (4oz) Medjool dates, chopped

50g (2oz) walnuts, chopped

250ML (8fl oz) milk

3 eggs

1 medium banana, mashed

1 tsp baking soda

Directions:

Sieve the baking soda and flour into a bowl.

Add in the banana, eggs, milk and dates and combine all the ingredients thoroughly.

Transfer the mixture to a lined loaf tin and smooth it out.

Scatter the walnuts on top.

Bake the loaf in the oven at 180C/360F for 45 minutes.

Transfer it to a wire rack to cool before serving.

Strawberry frozen yoghurt

Preparation time: 5 minutes | Cooking time: 0 minutes | Servings: 3

Ingredients:

450g (1Lb) plain yoghurt

175G (6oz) strawberries juice of

1 orange

1 tbsp honey

Directions:

Place the strawberries and orange juice into a food processor or blender and blitz until smooth.

Press the mixture through a sieve into a large bowl to remove seeds.

Stir in the honey and yoghurt.

Transfer the mixture to an ice-cream maker and follow the manufacturer's directions.

Alternatively pour the mixture into a container and place in the fridge for 1 hour.

Use a fork to whisk it and break up ice crystals and freeze for 2 hours.

Chocolate brownies

Preparation time: 5 minutes | Cooking time: 30 minutes | Servings: 3

Ingredients:

200g (7oz) dark chocolate (min 85% cocoa) 200g (7oz) Medjool dates, stone removed 100g (3½oz) walnuts, chopped 3 eggs

25ML (1fl oz) melted coconut oil 2 tsp vanilla essence ½ tsp baking soda

Makes 14 197 calories per serving

Directions:

Place the dates, chocolate, eggs, coconut oil, baking soda and vanilla essence into a food processor and mix until smooth.

Stir the walnuts into the mixture.

Pour the mixture into a shallow baking tray.

Transfer to the oven and bake at 180C/350F for 25-30 minutes.

Allow it to cool.

Cut into pieces and serve.

Crème brûlée

Preparation time: 5 minutes | Cooking time: 0 minutes | Servings: 3

Ingredients:

400g (14oz) strawberries

300g (11oz) plain low-fat yoghurt

125g (4oz) Greek yoghurt

100g (3½oz) brown sugar

1 tsp vanilla extract

Directions:

Divide the strawberries between 4 ramekin dishes.

In a bowl combine the plain yoghurt with the vanilla extract.

Spoon the mixture onto the strawberries. Scoop the Greek yoghurt on top.

Sprinkle the sugar into each ramekin dish, completely covering the top.

Place the dishes under a hot grill (broiler) for around 3 minutes or until the sugar has caramelised.

Pistachio fudge

Preparation time: 5 minutes | Cooking time: 0 minutes| Servings: 3

Ingredients:

225g (8oz) Medjool dates

100g (3½ oz) pistachio nuts, shelled (or other nuts)

50g (2oz) desiccated (shredded) coconut

25G (1oz) oats

2 tbsp water

Directions:

Place the dates, nuts, coconut, oats and water into a food processor and process until the ingredients are well mixed.

Remove the mixture and roll it to 2cm (1 inch) thick.

Cut it into 10 pieces and serve.

Spiced poached apples

Preparation time: 5 minutes | Cooking time: 0 minutes | Servings: 3

Ingredients:

4 apples

2 tbsp honey

4 star-anises

2 cinnamon sticks

300ml (½ pint) green tea

Directions:

Place the honey and green tea into a saucepan and bring to the boil.

Add the apples, star anise and cinnamon.

Reduce the heat and simmer gently for 15 minutes.

Serve the apples with a dollop of crème fraiche or Greek yoghurt.

Black forest smoothie

Preparation time: 5 minutes | Cooking time: 0 minutes | Servings: 3

Ingredients

100g (3½oz) frozen cherries

25G (1OZ) kale

1 Medjool date

1 tbsp cocoa powder

2 tsp chia seeds

200ml (7fl oz) milk or soya milk

Directions

Place all the ingredients into a blender and process until smooth and creamy.

Creamy coffee smoothie

Preparation time: 5 minutes | Cooking time: 0 minutes| Servings: 3

Ingredients:

1 banana

1 tsp chia seeds

1 tsp coffee

½ avocado

120ml (4fl oz) water

Serves 1

239 calories per serving

Directions:

Place all the ingredients into a food processor or blender and blitz until smooth.

You can add a little crushed ice too.

This can also double as a breakfast smoothie.

Grape and melon smoothie

Preparation time: 5 minutes | Cooking time: 0 minutes | Servings: 3

Ingredients:

100g of cantaloupe melon

100g of red seedless grapes

30g of young spinach leaves, stalks removed

½ cucumber

Directions:

Peel the cucumber, then cut it into half.

Remove the seeds and chop it roughly.

Peel the cantaloupe, deseed it, and cut it into chunks.

Place all ingredients in a blender and blend until smooth.

Sirt energy balls

Preparation time: 5 minutes | Cooking time: 40 minutes | Servings: 3

Ingredients:

1 mug of mixed nuts (with plenty of walnuts)

7 Medjool dates

1 tbsp of coconut oil

2 tbsp of cocoa powder

zest of 1 orange(optional)

Directions:

Start by placing the nuts in a food processor and grind them until almost powdered (more or less depending on the preferred texture of your energy balls).

Add the Medjool dates, coconut oil, cacao powder, and run the blender again until fully mixed.

Place the blend in a refrigerator for half an hour, and then shape them into balls.

You can add in the zest of an orange as you blend.

Cupcakes with matcha icing

Preparation time: 5 minutes | Cooking time: 50 minutes | Servings: 3

Ingredients:

½ tsp of salt

200g of caster sugar

½ tsp of vanilla extract

150G of self-rising flour

60g of cocoa

1 egg

120ml milk

½ tsp of fine espresso coffee, decaf if preferred

120ml of boiling water

50ml of vegetable oil

For the icing:

1 tbsp of matcha green tea powder

50g of at room temperature butter

50g of icing sugar

½ tsp of vanilla bean paste

50g of soft cream cheese

Directions:

Heat the oven to 160-180C fan.

Line a cupcake tin with silicone cake cases or paper.

Thoroughly mix salt, flour, cocoa, sugar, and espresso powder in a large bowl.

Add the milk, vegetable oil, vanilla extract, and egg to the other ingredients and beat them well using an electric mixer.

Carefully pour boiling water into the electric mixer and mix on low speed until perfectly combined.

Mix on high for about a minute to add some air into the batter.

The batter will appear liquid than what you would expect for normal cakes; this is how it should be.

Evenly add the batter into the cake cases no more than ¾ full.

Place them into the preheated oven and bake for about 15-18 minutes or until the mixture can bounce back when tapped.

When done, remove from the oven and allow them to cool before icing.

For the icing, mix the icing sugar and the butter until pale and smooth.

Add matcha powder mixed with vanilla and stir well again.

Finally, add the cream cheese and mix until smooth.

Spread this mixture over the cakes and serve.

Matcha juice

Preparation time: 5 minutes | Cooking time: 0 minutes| Servings: 3

Ingredients:

½ tsp of matcha powder (or you can use 1 tea bag strongly pre-steeped in a ¼ cup of water, and cooled)

2 handfuls of kale

Handful arugula

2-3 stalks of celery

½ granny smith (green, tart) apple

3 sprigs parsley

½ lemon, but juiced prior

Directions:

Juice the vegetables and fruit.

Squeeze the lemon in afterwards (do not juice it).

Stir in the matcha green tea powder or the chilled green tea afterwards.

Very green juice

Preparation time: 5 minutes | Cooking time: 0 minutes | Servings: 3

Ingredients:

1 kiwi, peeled, halved

½ cup pre-pressed apple juice

½ ripe pear, cored

1 cup baby spinach leaves (pull off stems if you would like)

¼ avocado, pitted and scooped out

Directions:

Simply juice until smooth.

Summer watermelon juice

Preparation time: 5 minutes | Cooking time: 0 minutes | Servings: 3

Ingredients:

½ cucumber, halved

2 cups baby kale (can remove stems if you like)

2 cups of pre-cut watermelon chunks

4 mint leaf

Directions:

Add all to a blender and blend it very well. Enjoy.

You cannot juice watermelon!

Banana berry smoothie

Preparation time: 5 minutes | Cooking time: 0 minutes | Servings: 3

Ingredients:

1 banana

1 cup blackberries

1 cup blueberries

2 tbsp natural yoghurt

1 cup milk (or soy/almond or rice milk)

Directions:

Add all to a blender and process until smooth.

Matcha green tea smoothie

Preparation time: 5 minutes | Cooking time: 0 minutes | Servings: 3

Ingredients:

2 bananas

2 tsp matcha green tea powder

½ tsp vanilla bean (paste or scraped from a vanilla bean pod)

1½ cups milk

4-5 ice cubes

2 tsp honey

Directions:

Add all ingredients except the matcha to a blender.

Blend until smooth.

Sprinkle in the matcha tea powder, stir well or blend a few seconds more (or add cooled green tea).

Green-berry smoothie

Preparation time: 5 minutes | Cooking time: 0 minutes | Servings: 3

Ingredients:

1 ripe banana

½ cup blackcurrants (take off stems)

10 baby kale leaves (take off stems)

2 tsp honey

1 cup freshly made green tea (dissolve honey first in tea then chill)

6 ice cubes

Directions:

Dissolve the honey in the tea before you chill it.

Cool first, and then blend all ingredients blender until smooth.

Green grapefruit smoothie

Preparation time: 5 minutes | Cooking time: 0 minutes | Servings: 3

Ingredients:

1 grapefruit, peeled and deseeded

6 large kale leaves, destemmed

1 green or red apple, cored and destemmed.

1 carrot

½ cup of water (may use more or less for the texture that you like)

Directions:

Place everything into a blender, and blend until smooth.

Add water if needed.

Green apple smoothie

Preparation time: 5 minutes | Cooking time: 0 minutes| Servings: 3

Ingredients:

1 green apple, cored and destemmed and sliced

6 large kale leaves, destemmed

1 orange, peeled

1 stick of celery

Directions:

Juice the orange separately in a blender and strain, unless you have a citrus juicer/press.

Juice the celery, kale and apple, mix together and stir, or add to a blender and pulse for a few seconds.

Creamy green sunshine smoothie

Preparation time: 5 minutes | Cooking time: 0 minutes | Servings: 3

Ingredients:

1 avocado, pitted and scooped out

1 banana

5 leaves of kale, destemmed

½ cup of pineapple juice

8 oz. of coconut water

Directions:

Place the liquids then the fruits and veggies into a blender and blend until smooth.

Pizza kale chips

Preparation time: 5 minutes| Cooking time: 40 minutes | Servings: 3

Ingredients:

250G (9oz) kale, chopped into approx. 4cm (2INch)

50g (2oz) ground almonds

50g (2oz) parmesan cheese

3 tbsp tomato purée (tomato paste)

½ tsp mixed herbs

½ tsp oregano

½ tsp onion powder

2 tbsp olive oil

100ml (3½ fl oz) water

Directions:

Place all of the ingredients, except the kale, into food processor and process until finely chopped into a smooth consistency.

Toss the kale leaves in the parmesan mixture, coating it really well.

Spread the kale out onto 2 baking sheets.

Bake in the oven at 170C/325F for 15 minutes, until crispy.

Rosemary & garlic kale chips

Preparation time: 5 minutes | Cooking time: 20 minutes | Servings: 3

Ingredients:

250G (9oz) kale chips, chopped into approx. 4cm (2inch)

2 sprigs of rosemary

2 cloves of garlic

2 tbsp olive oil sea salt

Freshly ground black pepper

Directions:

Gently warm the olive oil, rosemary and garlic over low heat for 10 minutes.

Remove it from the heat and set aside to cool.

Take the rosemary and garlic out of the oil and discard them.

Toss the kale leaves in the oil, making sure they are well coated.

Season with salt and pepper.

Spread the kale leaves onto 2 baking sheets and bake them in the oven at 170C/325F for 15 minutes, until crispy.

Chapter 9: Questions and Answers

What's the reason?

It depends on eating a gathering of nourishments that contain something the creators portray as 'sirtuin activators'. Sirtuins are a class of protein, seven of which (sirt1 to sirt7) have been recognized in people. They seem to have a wide scope of jobs in our body, including potential enemies of maturing and metabolic impacts.

As researchers see increasingly about sirtuins, they're getting keen on the job they may play in assisting with turning on those weight reduction pathways that are normally activated by an absence of nourishment and by taking activity. The hypothesis goes that in the event that you can actuate a portion of the seven sirtuins, you could assist with consuming fat and treat weight with less exertion than it takes to follow some different eating regimens or go through hours on the treadmill.

What does it include?

The sirtfood diet has two phases. On every one of the initial three days, you drink three 'sirt juices' and have one supper (aggregate of 1,000 calories per day). On the accompanying four days, you're permitted two sirt juices and two dinners day by day (aggregate of 1,500 calories day by day). You at that point progress to the simpler stage two, with one juice and three 'adjusted' dinners, in reasonable bit measures, a day.

What would you be able to eat on the eating regimen?

There's a rundown of nourishments containing synthetic intensifies that the creators' state switches on sirtuin and wrench up fat consumption while at the same time bringing down hunger (the last most likely through assisting with accomplishing better glucose control).

Is it compelling for weight reduction?

You ought to get in shape essentially on the grounds that you're eating fewer calories, particularly in stage one. Without a doubt, you may consume fat quicker with this eating routine than with 'any old calorie-confined' plan, and you may feel more full. With respect to the creators' case, this eating regimen is 'clinically demonstrated to lose 7lb in seven days'...

Indeed, it's important that so far the eating regimen has just been tried on 40 sound, exceptionally energetic human guinea pigs in an upmarket rec centre in London's

Knightsbridge. The analyzers lost a normal of 7lb in seven days while demonstrating increments in bulk and vitality. In any case, at that point, given the calorie limitations of that first week, weight reduction may essentially be because of the extraordinary decrease in calories.

Further examinations are expected to distinguish the long haul sway on waistlines – and general wellbeing – and to see whether sirt calorie counters keep the pounds off any more adequately than they would on different eating regimens. We don't yet have the foggiest idea what, assuming any, sway the expansion of sirt foods to our eating regimen really has on our weight.

What's more, will anybody have the option to stay with the repetitiveness of juices and limit themselves to nourishments on the rundown (and be glad to dump their typical cuppa for green tea) for all time? With respect to the features that recommend you can appreciate dull chocolate and red wine on this eating regimen – well, truly, it is anything but a green light to expend piles of either!

In the event that you have the funds, the tendency and the stomach for it, I'm very certain it will 'attempt' somewhat for the time being, if simply because it's a successful Directions to confine calories. Furthermore, wine and chocolate aside, the rundown, for the most part, comprises of the very nourishments dietitians and nutritionists suggest for good wellbeing (think products of the soil!).

Regardless of whether it functions admirably enough to make it stand separated from a huge number of weight reduction designs that have trodden this tired way before likewise is not yet clear.

Conclusion

The sirtfood diet promotes fat burning, body detoxification, muscle gain and overall health improvement by tapping into sirtuin, or in other words, activates your very own 'skinny gene'.

Though a relatively new diet, it is proven to be effective and yields fast and safe results. As a bonus, you can still eat chocolate and enjoy drinking wine!

I hope this book was able to help you find a suitable and effective diet regimen that will help you on your weight loss journey.

The next step is to continue what you have started, maintain your ideal weight and to choose to be healthy each day.

The first week might be a challenge for you, but as they say, if you want changes, you need to work for it. I guarantee you that once you start seeing the improvements in your body, you will realize that a little sacrifice is totally worth it.

In addition to the aesthetic changes that you will see, it is actually what is "inside" that really counts. Achieving optimum health is now possible with the numerous health benefits of the sirtfood diet. I promise you that the quality of your life will surely be improved, all it takes is adding those healthy sirtuin-rich foods!

Test out all of the recipes, and follow along with each of the phases with the proper foods and drinks. Follow the two planned stages, phase 1 and phase 2, and you will be guaranteed to enjoy more energy, vitality, a lighter feeling, and on average, about 7 lbs. Lighter on the scale each week.

THE SIRTFOOD DIET COOKBOOK

Over 200 easy, delicious recipes to start your new lifestyle and help you to lose up 7 LBS in 7 days. Discovered new super foods and their incredible benefits!

Adele Fung

Introduction

This book contains proven steps and strategies on how to not only follow the sirtfood diet but to really understand how and why it works.

Here's an inescapable fact: you will want a diet plan that you can not only use to lose weight perhaps. You will want one that you will find so delicious and so easy to follow that it can become a part of your life.

If you do not understand why a particular diet works or know how you can sustain it after the test period, you most likely will abandon all that you have learned. The other frustrating part of most diets is that most people will gain the weight back afterwards because they don't either know how or do not want to continue to maintain the new lifestyle. This diet is different.

It's time for you to become the most amazingly vital, youthful, and in shape person that you can be. We hope that you enjoy this book as we explore the benefits of the sirtfood diet!

Sounds unrealistic, we know, however with red wine and dim chocolate on the menu, the sirtfood diet as of now has armies of supporters and is set to overwhelm the eating regimen world.

The sirtfood diet has been hailed as the only diet that encourages you to include certain foods instead of just drastically reducing your calorie intake. The food inclusions are some of our favourite food, like chocolate!

It may seem too good to be true but let me assure you that this diet is purely scientific and has been tested by nutrition scientists Aidan Goggins and Glen Matten who are also the proponents of the diet. The duo also tested this food program at an upmarket gym in west London.

There are also a number of testimonies on the effectivity of the diet. To date, some of the followers of this diet are tv personalities/model Lorraine Pascale and Jodie Kidd, boxers Anthony Ogogo and David Haye, rugby player James Haskell and more. The Google searches for sirtfood diet has actually spiked since late 2015. In fact, this diet is predicted to become of the most popular diet this year.

The proponents have also stressed that this is not a fad diet; it is here to stay because not only does it promote weight loss, it can also boost your immune system and improve overall health.

And the good thing about sirtfoods? Since this is not a fad diet, you are free from the terrible bounce-back or yo-yo diet effect! It is easy to maintain and include in your regular diet, and there are hundreds of dishes or meals that you can do from the list. In addition, sirtfoods are easily available, there is no need for special meals, and it definitely won't break the bank. Coupled with regular exercise, you are on the way to achieving your better health and lose those extra pounds.

This book is the perfect companion to the official sirtfood diet book and provides you with over 200 easy and delicious recipes rich in sirtfoods to make your sirtfood diet meal planning a breeze.

Best wishes with your new diet. I hope you enjoy it!

Chapter 1: What are the sirtfoods?

The sirtfood diet was created by UK nutritionists Aidan Goggins and Glen Matten, who distributed a top-rated book on the point in 2016. It vows to lessen irritation, lengthen your life range, turn on your "thin quality" and assist you with shedding seven pounds (three kilograms) in seven days. It asserts that eating specific nourishments will interface with a gathering of proteins found in the body called sirtuins (sirts), which are engaged with a wide scope of cell forms including digestion, maturing and circadian cadence.

Beside expending a scope of "sirtfoods," the diet includes phases of calorie limitation, which is likewise said to enable the body to create more sirtuins. During the initial three says calorie admission is restricted to 1,000 every day, sourced from three green juices and sirtfood-rich dinner. For the remainder of the week, calorie admission is helped to 1,500 every day from two juices and two dinners. The subsequent stage keeps going 14 days and prompts three adjusted sirtfood rich suppers daily alongside one sirtfood green juice. Long haul its advocates suggest eating suppers with however many sirtfoods as could reasonably be expected.

There are many sirtuin-activating foods to choose from, with some containing more sirtuin-activating ingredients than others. These we have called the 'top sirtfoods', and these foods are included in all of our recipes, to maximise your sirtfood intake.

It has gotten the most loved of big names in Europe and is popular for permitting red wine and chocolate.

Its makers demand that it is anything but a prevailing fashion, yet rather than "sirtfoods" are the key to opening fat misfortune and forestalling malady.

In any case, wellbeing specialists caution that this eating routine may not satisfy everyone's expectations and could even be a poorly conceived notion.

Two VIP nutritionists working for a private rec centre in the UK built up the sirtfood diet.

They publicize the eating regimen as a progressive new eating regimen and wellbeing plan that works by turning on your "thin quality."

This eating regimen depends on investigating on sirtuins (sirts), a gathering of seven proteins found in the body that has been appeared to manage an assortment of capacities, including digestion, irritation and life expectancy certain characteristic plant mixes might have the option to build the degree of these proteins in the body, and nourishments containing them have been named "sirtfoods."

The sirtfood diet depends on look into on sirtuins, a gathering of proteins that direct a few capacities in the body. Certain nourishments called sirtfoods may make the body produce a greater amount of these proteins.

Is it effective?

The creators of the sirtfood diet make intense cases, including that the eating regimen can super-charge weight reduction, turn on your "thin quality" and forestall sicknesses.

The issue is there isn't a lot of confirmation to back them.

Up until this point, there's no persuading proof that the sirtfood diet has a more helpful impact on weight reduction than some other calorie-limited eating routine.

Furthermore, albeit a considerable lot of these nourishments have restorative properties, there have not been any long haul human investigations to decide if eating an eating routine rich in sirtfoods has any substantial medical advantages.

By and by, the sirtfood diet book reports the aftereffects of a pilot study directed by the writers and including 39 members from their wellness focus. In any case, the aftereffects of this examination show up not to have been distributed anyplace else.

For the multi-week, the members followed the eating regimen and practised every day. Toward the week's end, members lost a normal of 7 pounds (3.2 kg) and kept up or even picked up the bulk.

However, these outcomes are not really amazing. Confining your calorie admission to 1,000 calories and practising simultaneously will about consistently cause weight reduction.

Notwithstanding, this sort of speedy weight reduction is neither authentic nor durable, and this investigation didn't follow members after the primary week to check whether they restored any of the weight, which is normally the situation.

At the point when your body is vitality denied, it goes through its crisis vitality stores, or glycogen, notwithstanding consuming fat and muscle.

Every atom of glycogen requires 3–4 particles of water to be put away. At the point when your body goes through glycogen, it disposes of this water too. It's known as "water weight."

In the principal seven day stretch of extraordinary calorie limitation, just around 33% of the weight reduction originates from fat, while the other 66% originates from water, muscle, and glycogen.

When your calorie admission expands, your body recharges its glycogen stores, and the weight returns right.

Sadly, this sort of calorie limitation can likewise make your body bring down its metabolic rate, causing you to need significantly fewer calories every day for vitality than previously.

Almost certainly, this eating regimen may assist you with shedding a couple of pounds first and foremost, yet it will probably return when the eating routine is finished.

To the extent of forestalling sickness, three weeks is presumably not long enough to have any quantifiable long haul sway.

Then again, adding sirtfoods to your normal eating routine over the long haul might just be a smart thought. Be that as it may, all things considered, you should skirt the eating regimen and start doing that now.

This eating regimen may assist you with getting more fit since it is low in calories, yet the weight is probably going to return once the eating routine closures. The eating routine is too short to even think about having a long haul sway on your wellbeing.

The most effective **Directions:** to follow the sirtfood diet

The sirtfood diet has two stages that last a sum of three weeks. From that point onward, you can keep "certifying" your eating routine by including, however many sirtfoods as could be allowed in your suppers.

Medical advantages of sirtfood diet

Sirtfood diet diminishes the danger of heart infections, heftiness, diabetes, and early demise. Individuals who are following this eating regimen plan has encountered a few medical advantages, generally safe of ailment and prosperity. As indicated by the diary, advances in nutrition composed by prof. Straight to the point hu, sirtfood diet assists with improving memory, oversee blood glucose levels and forestall oxidative worry in the body. A portion of the regular medical advantages of sirtfood counts calories are as per the following:

It will assist you with losing fat, not muscles.

- the eating routine won't deplete your vitality and rather keep you increasingly lively.
- as it thoroughly relies upon diet, setting off to the rec centre or performing thorough activities is a bit much.
- the eating regimen plan stays away from the self-starvation hypothesis for weight reduction.
- it forestalls various ceaseless illnesses as the nourishments remembered for this eating regimen plan are solid and nutritive.

Who should try sirtfood diet?

Are you familiar with these scenarios?

You know that you have overindulged during the holidays, but as you weigh yourself, you literally would want to shave all the extra pounds because you did not expect to have gained that much weight!

There is an upcoming wedding event, and you need to lose those extra pounds in order to fit yourself into your gown/suit. There is no way that you are going to lose that much weight in 2 months!

You know that you are overweight and just plain unhealthy. You have already tried a number of diets but to no avail. Either you feel that those diets are too restrictive, there is an adverse health effect, and the diet is too expensive to maintain. Speaking of maintenance, you have a hard time to keep off the little weight that you have managed to lose!

You are getting older, and you start to notice that aside from having a hard time dealing with hangovers and late-night parties, losing and maintaining weight is not that easy as it used to be. You are not a big fan of eliminating numerous food groups and doing rigorous exercise.

You have probably heard these scenarios too many times before, and you have probably experienced one or two, or you are in one of these scenarios right now. Being overweight or obese is actually one of the most common health problems around the world. According to the world health organization (who), being overweight is when your BMI is equal to or greater than 25 while being obese is when your BMI is equal to or greater than 30 (you can check your BMI **here**.)

In the 2014 data from who, worldwide obesity has more than doubled since 1980, and more than 1.9 billion adults are overweight; and it would be safe to conclude that after two years that that number has already increased significantly.

Health experts agree that this is a very alarming rate, but the good news is, obesity or having excess weight is preventable and reversible.

As you will notice, most of these scenarios are focused on the aesthetics – looking good and feeling more confident about your body, but what i would like to stress is the ill-effects of every extra bulge or pound that we carry. The possible health illnesses associated with being overweight is the primary reason why you need to try the revolutionary sirtfood diet.

Health risks for overweight and obesity

Type 2 diabetes - this disease occurs when the blood sugar level becomes higher than the normal. According to studies, about 80% of individuals afflicted with type 2 diabetes are overweight. What makes diabetes a killer disease is that it is a major cause of stroke, heart disease, kidney diseases, amputation, and even blindness.

Sleep apnea - this is when an individual pauses in breathing while sleeping. Being overweight or obese is a risk factor. Why? This is because of the fats stored in the neck area, making the air pathway smaller. In addition, the fat could also cause inflammation. Sleep apnea should not be taken lightly because it can also result in heart failure.

High blood pressure - also known as hypertension, this condition refers to a state when your systolic blood pressure (usually above 140) is consistently higher than your diastolic blood pressure (usually about 90). How does being overweight make you 'high risk' for hypertension? Generally, larger body size will increase your blood pressure so that your heart will have to work harder to produce the necessary supply of blood to all cells. In addition, your excess body fats can damage your kidneys (your kidney helps your body regulate the blood pressure). High blood pressure can result in kidney failure, heart diseases and stroke.

Fatty liver disease - this is when there is a build-up of fat around the liver which can cause damage.

Reproductive issues - menstrual issues and infertility are some of the issues experienced by overweight women.

Cancer - if you are obese or overweight, then the risk of acquiring cancer of the breast, gallbladder, colon and endometrial increases.

These are only some of the diseases associated with being overweight; not to mention the social, emotional and psychological impact of the extra weight.

It stresses the importance of finding the right "strategy" to lose those excess pounds. And we have the perfect solution –the sirtfood diet.

The sirtfood diet is suitable for individuals who:

- Are overweight or obese
- Want to maintain his/her weight
- Needs to have a "detox" and flush away the toxins from the body
- Have failed to lose weight using different diet techniques
- Want not only to lose weight but also build muscle
- Want a healthier lifestyle and to achieve optimal health

Shopping

Now that you have decided on a juicer let us look at some of the common sirtfoods that are included in the recipes that were listed earlier, and try to make it easier to prepare. If you can, try to buy fresh, and also organic. Locations may vary, and some things may be purchased bulk. These are some of the top sirtfoods, and the top-top super sirtfoods (with an asterisk*). There are more than are on this list, but these will be the most common ones and the ones that will be mostly used in this book. You can do a Google search and research other sirtfoods after you get the hang of the plan. Also, see the section on sirtfood diet phases, where you are encouraged to do the plan now and at any time in the future, in addition to staying in the maintenance phase, you can go back to phases 1 and 2. You can get creative, use these or the different sirtfoods, and rev up your metabolism again as you would like!

apples
arugula
blackcurrants*
buckwheat
capers* dates (Medjool)
celery
chicory (red)
citrus fruits-oranges, grapefruits

cocoa (dark chocolate, 85% or more)*

coffee

extra virgin olive oil

fish oil (omega-3)*

green tea (matcha preferable)*

kale*

lovage

miso soup, and other soy products

olives*

onions (red)*

parsley*

red wine

strawberries

tofu

turmeric*

walnuts

Cooking with sirtfoods

Now that you have read the list of sirtfoods, it's time to plan your menu so that you can shop for all your required ingredients. If possible, aim to buy your fresh ingredients every few days and include sirtfoods in every meal.

By far, the best way to load up on those sirtfoods is to start your day with a healthy smoothie. Especially a green one as it's a great refreshing kick start to your body and you can easily pack in 5Fruits/vegetables in one drink. It's sure to keep hunger away too!

We've provided lots of recipes for smoothies which you can not only have for breakfast but as a lunch replacement or mid-day snack. Bear in mind that although the recipes have been categorised as breakfast, light bites and main meals etc. You are free to swap them around.

If you have had a busy day and haven't been able to pack in the sirt goodies as much as you would like, you can always supplement with a handful of walnuts, a green tea or a coffee in between meals to give you a boost and keep hunger away.

If you are careful with your calorie intake, you can be guided by the information on each recipe. A little word of caution when it comes to dates or 'nature's toffees' as some people call them – they are rich in calories. One date contains around 61 calories, so don't go overboard. That said, if you would normally reach for cakes, sweets or biscuits then a date or two is a good substitute because you won't be consuming empty refined sugar calories, yet still enjoying a sweet treat.

If you haven't already, swap your normal cuppa for green tea which has virtually zero calories. If you don't have a taste for it, you can try it with a flavouring such as jasmine, or even try the recipe for iced cranberry green tea for a refreshing way to drink it. Matcha, which is a type of green tea, is an even stronger tea which also comes in a powder which can be added to smoothies and cooking. Health shops stock matcha, or alternatively, you can buy it online.

Keep a parsley plant on your window ledge because you can add it to virtually anything or even nibble on a sprig! Lovage is a relative of parsley, which has even greater sirtuin-activating benefits, so if you can find it (and it's a big if) use that instead of parsley. Because it's not so easy to find, we have not included lovage in any of these recipes, but if you do get hold of some just add it in.

Capers are available in most supermarkets and sold in jars. They do have a strong salty flavour so you won't need to use too many.

When it comes to chocolate, don't be tempted to buy a sugar-laden milk chocolate bar at the check-out because it won't contain much cocoa. Always aim for good quality dark chocolate with a high cocoa content of around 85% cocoa. Yes, it is more bitter, but your taste buds will soon adapt, and a square of chocolate after a meal is a great treat to round off the day.

The eating regimen originates from the book of a similar name. The creators – Aidan Goggins and Glen Matten – of the sirtfood diet exhort eating for the most part nourishments rich in sirtuins, a sort of protein in plant nourishments. "The eating plan itself is intended to 'turn on' the sirtuin qualities (especially sirt-1), which are accepted to support digestion, increment fat consuming, battle aggravation, and control craving," says Clark.

Early investigations propose that calorie limitation and resveratrol (a polyphenol found in nourishments like grapes, blueberries, and peanuts), initiate the sirt-1 quality, and these two standards support the sirtfood way to deal with eating.

Chapter 2: How to follow the sirtfood diet

In the realm of diet and nourishment, there's constantly another approach to shed pounds. The most recent technique, upheld by any semblance of Pippa Middleton and Adele, was laid out in detail not long ago in a book called the sirtfood diet, which gives a sustenance plan based on nourishments like kale, green tea, dim chocolate, wine, blueberries, olive oil, soy, and different food sources high in specific plant exacerbates that invigorate proteins called sirtuins.

"Sirtuins are a class of proteins found in living things" – including people – "that exploration has demonstrated to be engaged with significant organic procedures, for example, maturing, cell demise, aggravation, and digestion," says Stacy Sims, PhD, a games nourishment master and senior research individual at the Adams centre for high performance at the University of Waikato in New Zealand.

As such, sirtuins may assist you with living longer, and according to their advocates, they may likewise assist you with shedding muscle versus fat. The expectation is that eating a huge amount of sirtfoods will invigorate the sirtuin qualities (at times called thin qualities) along these lines to fasting. Yet, does it truly work that way? To begin with, some foundation: in well-evolved creatures, there are seven kinds of sirtuins, which extend from sirt1 to sirt7. of them, sirt1 is the one that analysts are generally keen on, says Sims. "sirt1 is some of the time alluded to as the 'gatekeeper' against oxidative pressure and DNA harm."

The possibility of the sirtfood diet is if you can actuate sirt1, you can create more mitochondria, the powerhouse of the cells, which will help diminish oxidative pressure, permitting you to age slower, says Mike Roussell, PhD, a dietary advisor in Philadelphia.

The issue? "You can't in any way, shape or form devour enough of the nourishments prescribed by this diet to increment sirtuins," says Roussell. Take red wine, which is remembered for the sirtfood diet: "to get 20 milligrams of resveratrol [a cancer prevention agent that invigorates sirt1], you would need to drink in excess of 40 glasses of wine," Roussell says. Which, all things considered, we aren't proposing you do.

Additionally, inquire about from endocrine journal finds that sirt1 directs craving differently from individual to individual. "so for certain individuals, expanded sirt1 articulation may make you hungry," says Roussell.

Presently, the way that individuals get more fit by following the sirtfood diet likely boils down to two elements:

The nourishments in the arrangement will, in general, be wealthy in supplements.

The book requires seven days of exceptional calorie limitation – only 1,000 calories every day for the initial three days and 1,500 per day for the remainder of the week. Furthermore, the vast majority of those calories are from juice.

Confining calories, as you presumably know, is the most dependable system for getting in shape. What's more, for what it's worth, inquire about from Finland's Helsinki University found that low-calorie diets may normally increment sirtuin action, whether or not you're eating sirtuin-rich nourishments or not.

So sure, add a couple of sirtuin nourishments to your diet: kale, strawberries, pecans, buckwheat, celery, red onions – all great stuff. Be that as it may, don't expect that you can't eat whatever else. If you're not kidding about getting thinner, centre around lean protein, vegetables, and entire grains – and hold your all-out vitality admission down.

Medical advantages of tailing it:

Just as helping you feel invigorated, the sirtuin activators can help direct your digestion, increment muscle and consume fat, according to Goggins and Matten.

Symptoms:

The writers guarantee that the objective of the sirt diet is more about good dieting than sensational weight loss, yet a few nutritionists have protested the way that their book is embellished with the slogan "lose 7lbs in 7 days". A loss of 1 to 2Lbs seven days is viewed as a relentless and solid sum. So such sensational weight loss in a brief period may not be useful for your prosperity. Additionally, self-evident, however important: red wine is loaded with poisons, regardless of whether it is high in sirtuin activators, so swallowing it as a feature of a 'diet' presumably is definitely not a smart thought. Darn.

According to the book's slogan, there is potential for fast transient weight loss. This depends on an exacting arrangement, including calorie control – 1,000 the initial three days, then increasing this to 1,500 – and expending a set quantities of green juices and sirtfood-rich suppers. In any case, in the long haul, the objective is essential to eat whatever number sirtfoods as could be allowed.

Sirtfood meal plans

When you follow the sirtfood diet, you'll start with stage 1 – which goes on for seven days. During the initial three days of the diet, you'll drink three sirtfood squeezes and have one sirtfood-rich dinner for a day by day aggregate of 1,000 calories. On days four however through seven you'll devour 1,500 complete calories, drink two green squeezes and eat two solid sirtfood-rich suppers. This finishes stage 1.

Stage 2 endures 14 days and permits you to eat three adjusted sirtfood-rich dinners and one green squeeze every day. After stage 2 is finished, you'll follow a progressively ordinary **Directions:** for eating – however, are urged to fuse sirtuin-actuating nourishments into normal supper plans. You can return stage 1 and 2 whenever you have to lose more weight or muscle to fat ratio.

Does the diet work?

Scientists analyzed the impacts of sirtfoods (sirtuin-enacting nourishments) on wellbeing and weight the board. One 2013 investigation found that diets rich in sirtfoods seem to help with sound maturing and constant ailment avoidance. A 2017 audit presumed that polyphenols seem to assist lower with bodying weight, blood glucose, and circulatory strain – however, more research is required around there.

One explanation you'll likely shed pounds if you follow the sirtfood diet accurately is on the grounds that you'll decrease calories (at any rate in stage 1) to 1,000 to 1,500 calories for each day, which is a nearly surefire approach to drop weight.

The primary concern is while you don't need to eat sirtuin-actuating nourishments to shed pounds (just bringing down your general calorie admission ought to work), most of the sirtfoods are sound, seem to bring down ailment dangers, and help in solid weight the board.

These thin pathways are similar ones all the more regularly initiated by fasting and exercise and help the body to consume fat, to build bulk and improve your wellbeing.

Nations where individuals as of now expend countless sirtfoods as a component of their customary diet, including Japan and Italy, are both routinely positioned among the most beneficial nations on the planet.

Aidan and Glen have quite recently discharged their book; the sirtfood diet – the progressive arrangement for wellbeing and weight loss.

Sirtfoods animate sirtuin qualities, which are said to impact the body's capacity to consume fat and lift the metabolic framework.

Follow these stages

Stage one is a serious seven-day program intended to launch your exceptional weight loss. Then stage two is tied in with increasing the amount of sirtfood-rich produce in your ordinary dinners to keep up weight loss.

Dissimilar to numerous other present moment yo-yo diets, the sirtfood plan remembers suppers and guidance for how to keep off the weight you lose in the main week by proceeding to incorporate sirtfoods as a feature of a sound and adjusted diet.

What does a commonplace day resemble?

Stage one

You can have 15-20g of dim chocolate after your feast if you have a sweet tooth.

For the second 50% of your first week, you can have two juices and two suppers every day, with comparable fixings to the initial three days.

Stage two

After the underlying phase of fasting the centre shifts to eating 'ordinarily' once more, however, increasing your admission of the sound sirtfoods. Continue perusing for Aidan and Glen's first-class sirtfood fixings!

Who is it useful for?

In spite of the fact that the underlying phase of squeezing and fasting just appears to be useful for the individuals who should shift a couple of pounds rapidly, the general frame of mind of the sirtfood diet is to incorporate more beneficial nourishments into your diet to build your prosperity and lift your resistant framework after some time.

So while the initial seven days appear to be no-nonsense, the more drawn out term plan works for everybody.

What are the cons?

The primary seven day stretch of the arrangement is truly in-your-face. Days one to three are generally escalated with your calorie admission restricted to 1,000 – consolidated of three juices and one dinner.

Days four to seven are somewhat more indulgent with a calorie limit of 1,500 calories for each day.

Aidan and Glen express that so as to battle the fasting time frame, don't concentrate on how much weight you are losing, rather take a gander at the wellbeing sway on your tone and how your garments fit, also how brilliant your skin will look.

Video of the week

Sirtfood diet phases

The sirtfood diet has two unique phases designed to do what you have learned sirtuins will trigger the body to do. It is a fourteen-day plan broken up into two phases, where each of the foods or drinks will have their place.

You will start with a lower amount of calories and then gradually increase them. This will jump-start your genes and trigger, by way of the sirtfoods, the sirtuin proteins to do their job on your "skinny genes."

Phase 1 – 1,000 calories

Days 1-3

1. 3 green juices
2. 1 cooked sirtfood meal (sirt)

Your calories each day of this phase should not go over 1,000. This is your reset button.

Days 4-7

1. 2 green juices
2. 2 cooked sirtfood meals

Your calories each day of this phase should not go over 1,500. If followed properly, this phase reports a 7lb Weight loss on average each week.

Phase 2 – 1,500 calories

This is a 14-day maintenance plan whereby you do not focus on restricting calories, but you must have at least one green juice. The rest are sirt meals.

This diet is unlike other diets where it does not end; it truly becomes a part of your lifestyle and could be a permanent way of eating. There would be no restrictions after the traditional diet has ended.

To begin the first phase, simply follow the directions in the getting started on sirtfoods chapter.

- purchase your food items based off of the recipes that you think you will like.
- some of the foods will become staples, so you may always want to keep them around.
- prepare how you will juice.
- plan when you will cook, including planning around being away from home or work.

When you get past phase 2, you can eat from sirtfoods as you please. The other great thing about the sirtfood diet is that you can go back to phases 1 and 2 at any time. You have the tools, and you will have the recipes. You will also feel more confident about creating your own recipes using a variety of sirtfoods.

7 pounds in seven days

Phase: 1

Sirtfood diet: a diet plan which will help you lose weight in just 7 days

The sirtfood diet plan is partitioned into two simple stages. In the main stage, you need to confine your calorie admission to 1,000 cal/day for the initial three days, which will incorporate three sirtfood green juices and a one-time feast loaded up with sirtfoods. In the initial three days, an individual may feel hungry however from the fourth to the seventh day the starvation may somewhat go down as the individual may expand the calorie admission from 1,000 to 1,500 cal/day. This will incorporate two sirtfood green juices and two suppers every day. To plan green juices, individuals may pick from celery, kale, green tea, and parsley while for suppers, chicken, kale curry, prawns fry, turkey and buckwheat will be the best alternatives.

The second period of sirtfood is really when weight reduction begins to occur. This stage takes 14 days in which an individual expends three sirtfood-rich dinners every day alongside an extraordinary green juice. This assists with shedding seven pounds in seven days. Both the periods of the eating routine are planned on the plan to eat the sound and nutritive nourishments what nature offers.

The primary guideline behind the sirtfood diet is that it enacts the fat-decreasing procedure in the body alongside advancing bulk development. In any case, the inquiry that emerges in everybody's brain in the wake of realizing the initial two stages is what really occurs after the third seven day stretch of the eating regimen?

All things considered, the possibility of sirtfood diet is that it is for the individuals who truly adored the initial two periods of the eating routine and need to proceed in a good dieting way. Sirtfood diet isn't just about counting calories for those three weeks; however, picking this eating routine arrangement as a lifestyle. This eating routine arrangement is so compelling and solid that individuals who have seen the outcomes will clearly be urged to keep drinking green squeezes each day and incorporate sirtfood in their suppers. Regardless of whether, holding fast to this eating routine arrangement is unimaginable consistently, simply having solid nourishment and including a touch of sirtfood, the top will do incredible advantage to your body.

As indicated by a pilot study directed by Aidan and Glen, a specialist in a healthful prescription drug store, it is demonstrated that individuals have lost around 7lbs in 7 days with no abatement in their bulk. Those individuals have likewise revealed an expansion in their vitality, better rest and improvement of their skin.

Maintenance dill

Phase : 2

Attempting to look for some new year inspiration? All things considered, simply admire vocalist Adele's change and it will be all the inspiration you need. Aside from assisting with weight reduction, the eating regimen is additionally picking up prevalence since it permits red wine and chocolate. These proteins have been appeared to manage digestion, life expectancy, aggravation, and other substantial capacities.

While the guarantee of moment weight reduction and gigantic outcomes might be engaging, some prevailing fashion abstains from food seriously confine nutritional categories leaving you.

Following are probably the most popular sirtfoods:

Morning walk benefits: had a terrible day? Feeling low? Need to get thinner? Simply take a stroll outside! Here are the numerous advantages of morning strolls that will get you on your feet.

They guarantee that following this eating regimen will prompt brisk weight reduction, while likewise keeping up bulk and offering assurance from maladies.

The eating regimen has two stages, every one of which keeps going for three weeks. From that point forward, you can incorporate the same number of sirtfoods in your eating regimen in your dinners as you wish. Studies state that this eating routine can assist you with losing around 3 kilos in seven days' time.

Sirtfood diet can assist you with losing 3 kilos in seven days' time

In the event that you see the rundown of sirtfoods, they incorporate nourishments that can be effectively found in your kitchen.

Stage one of the sirtfood diet goes on for a time of 7 days. During the initial multi-day, you have to limit your calories to 1,000 calories. You have to drink 3 green juices and one feast. Sirtfoodomelete, shrimp pan-fried food, and buckwheat rot are a couple of alternatives you can attempt.

On the following 4 days of stage one, you can build your calorie consumption by up to 1,500 calories. You can have two green squeezes in a day alongside at least two sirtfood-rich suppers. Suppers can be set up by utilizing flexible sirtfoods.

Stage two of the sirtfood diet goes on for about fourteen days. This stage is otherwise called the upkeep period of sirtfood diet. You being to consistently shed pounds in this stage. There are no calorie restrictions you have to follow in this stage. You can have full three dinners and one glass of green squeeze in a day.

On the off chance that you need to, you can rehash the two stages, so as to arrive at your ideal weight. The eating routine can surely be your way of life rather than a one-time diet you took in the mood for getting more fit.

Chapter 3: Understanding sirtuins

Sirtuins help control your cell wellbeing. This is what you have to think about how they work, what they can accomplish for your body, and why they depend on nad+ to work.

How sirtuins regulate cellular health with nad+

Think about your body's cells like an office. In the workplace, there are numerous individuals working on different undertakings with an extreme objective: remain gainful and satisfy the strategic the organization in a proficient way for whatever length of time that conceivable. In the cells, there are numerous pieces working on different undertakings with an extreme objective, as well: remain solid and capacity proficiently for whatever length of time that conceivable. Similarly, as needs in the organization change, because of different inner and outside components, so do needs in the cells. Somebody needs to run the workplace, controlling what completes when, who will do it and when to switch course. In the workplace, that would be your CEO. In the body, at the cell level, it's your sirtuins.

Sirtuins are proteins. I'm not catching that's meaning?

Sirtuins are a group of proteins. Protein may seem like dietary protein – what's found in beans and meats and well, protein shakes – yet for this situation we're discussing particles called proteins, which work all through the body's phones in various different capacities. Consider proteins the divisions at an organization, everyone concentrating without anyone else specific capacity while planning with different offices.

Sirtuins work with acetyl bunches by doing what's called deacetylation. This implies they perceive there's an acetyl bunch on a particle then evacuate the acetyl gathering, which tees up the atom for its activity. One way that sirtuins work is by expelling acetyl gatherings (deacetylating) natural proteins, for example, histones. For instance, sirtuins deacetylate histones, proteins that are a piece of a dense type of DNA called chromatin. The histone is an enormous cumbersome protein that the DNA folds itself over. Consider it a Christmas tree, and the DNA strand is the strand of lights. When the histones have an acetyl gathering, the chromatin is open or loosened up.

This loosened up chromatin implies the DNA is being interpreted, a basic procedure. Yet, it doesn't have to remain loosened up, as it's defenceless against harm in this position, practically like the Christmas lights could get tangled or the bulbs can get harmed when they're awkward or up for a really long time. When the histones are deacetylated by sirtuins, the chromatin is shut, or firmly and perfectly twisted, which means quality articulation is halted or quieted.

We've just thought about sirtuins for around 20 years, and their essential capacity was found during the 1990s. From that point forward, specialists have rushed to examine them, identifying their significance while likewise bringing up issues about what else we can find out about them.

Activation the sirtuins

Sirtuins are a group of proteins that manage cell wellbeing. Sirtuins assume a key job in controlling cell homeostasis.

In the workplace, there are numerous individuals taking a shot at different assignments with an extreme objective: remain gainful and satisfy the strategic the organization in a productive way for whatever length of time that conceivable. In the cells, there are numerous pieces taking a shot at different undertakings with an extreme objective, as well: remain sound and capacity proficiently for whatever length of time that conceivable. Similarly, as needs in the organization change, because of different inside and outer variables, so do needs in the cells. Somebody needs to run the workplace, directing what completes when, who will do it and when to switch course.

Nad+ is essential to cell digestion and many other organic procedures. In the event that sirtuins are an organization's CEO, at that point, nad+ is the cash that pays the pay of the CEO and workers, all while keeping the lights on and the workplace space lease paid. An organization, and the body, can't work without it.

Protein may seem like dietary protein – what's found in beans and meats and well, protein shakes – yet for this situation we're discussing atoms called proteins, which work all through the body's phones in various capacities. Consider proteins the divisions at an organization, everyone concentrating without anyone else explicit capacity while planning with different offices.

Acetyl bunches control explicit responses. They're physical labels on proteins that different proteins perceive will respond with them. In the event that proteins are the branches of the cell and DNA is the CEO, the acetyl bunches are the accessibility status of every division head. For instance, in the event that a protein is accessible, at that point, the sirtuin can work with it to get something going, similarly as the CEO can work with an accessible division head to get something going.

Sirtuins work with acetyl bunches by doing what's called deacetylation. One way that sirtuins work is by evacuating acetyl gatherings (deacetylating) organic proteins, for example, histones. The histone is an enormous cumbersome protein that the DNA folds itself over. This loosened up chromatin implies the DNA is being translated, a fundamental procedure.

We've just thought about sirtuins for around 20 years, and their essential capacity was found during the 1990s. From that point forward, specialists have rushed to examine them, recognizing their significance while likewise bringing up issues about what else we can find out about them.

The discovery and history of sirtuins

In 1991, Elysium fellow benefactor and MIT scientist Leonard Guarente, close by graduate understudies Nick Austriaco and Brian Kennedy, directed tests to all the more likely see how yeast matured. By some coincidence, Austriaco attempted to develop societies of different yeast strains from tests he had put away in his ice chest for quite a long time, which made an unpleasant situation for the strains.

This is the place acetyl bunches become possibly the most important factor. It was at first idea that siR2 might be a deacetylating protein – which means it expelled those acetyl gatherings – from different atoms, however, nobody knew whether this was valid since all endeavours to show this movement in a test tube demonstrated negative.

In Guarente's very own words: "without nad+, siR2 sits idle. That was the basic finding on the circular segment of sirtuin science."

Fighting fat through sirtuins

Ecological factors significantly influence the destiny of living beings and sustenance is one of the most persuasive variables. These days life span is a significant objective of medicinal science and has consistently been a fabrication for the individual since antiquated occasions. Specifically, endeavours are planned for accomplishing effective maturing, to be specific a long life without genuine ailments, with a decent degree of physical and mental autonomy and satisfactory social connections.

Gathering information unmistakably exhibits that it is conceivable to impact the indications of maturing. Without a doubt, wholesome mediations can advance wellbeing and life span. A tribute must be given to Ancel Keys, who was the first to give strong logical proof about the job of sustenance in the wellbeing/sickness balance at the populace level, explicitly in connection to cardiovascular illness, still the main source of death overall. It is commonly valued that the sort of diet can significantly impact the quality and amount of life and the Mediterranean eating regimen is paradigmatic of an advantageous dietary example the developing cognizance of the useful impacts of a particular dietary example on wellbeing and life span in the second 50% of the only remaining century produced a ground-breaking push toward structuring eats fewer carbs that could diminish the danger of constant maladies, subsequently bringing about solid maturing. Subsequently, during the 1990s, the dietary approaches to stop hypertension (dash) diet was contrived so as to assess whether it was conceivable to treat hypertension, not pharmacologically. To be sure, the dash diet was very like the Mediterranean diet, being wealthy in foods grown from the ground, entire grains, and strands, while poor in creature soaked fats and cholesterol. The awesome news leaving the investigation was that not exclusively did the dash diet lower circulatory strain; however, it additionally diminished the danger of cardiovascular infection, type 2 diabetes, a few sorts of malignant growth, and other maturing related maladies to additionally improve the medical advantages of plant nourishment rich, creature fat-terrible eating routines, especially in hypercholesterolemic people, the portfolio diet was planned this eating regimen, other than being to a great extent veggie-lover, with just limited quantities of soaked fats, prescribes a high admission of utilitarian nourishments, including thick filaments, plant stanols, soy proteins, and almonds likewise. Curiously, members on the portfolio diet displayed a decrease of coronary illness chance related to lower plasma cholesterol and incendiary files in contrast with members on a sound, for the most part, vegan diet.

Nonetheless, additionally, the measure of ingested nourishment has been pulling in light of a legitimate concern for mainstream researchers as a potential modifier of the harmonyamong wellbeing and infection in a wide range of living species. Specifically, calorie limitation (cr) has been exhibited to be a rising healthful intercession that animates the counter maturing instruments in the body.

In this way, the eating routine of the individuals living on the Japanese island of Okinawa has been widely broken down on the grounds that these islanders are notable for their life span and expanded wellbeing range, bringing about the best recurrence of centenarians on the planet. Interestingly, the customary Okinawan diet came about to be fundamentally the same as the Mediterranean diet and the dash diet regarding nourishment types. Be that as it may, the vitality admission of Okinawans, at the hour of the underlying logical perceptions, was about 20% lower than the normal vitality admission of the Japanese, along these lines deciding an average state of cr.

In his most recent examination, showing up in the aug8 print release of the diary cell metabolism, he saw what happens when the sirt1 protein is absent from fat cells, which make up muscle versus fat.

At the point when putting on a high-fat eating regimen, mice coming up short on the protein began to create metabolic issues, for example, diabetes, much sooner than typical mice were given a high-fat eating routine.

"you've expelled one of the protections against metabolic decay, so on the off chance that you presently give them the trigger of a high-fat eating routine, they're considerably more delicate than the typical mouse."

The discovery raises the likelihood that medications that upgrade sirt1 action may help ensure against weight connected illnesses. From that point forward, these proteins have been appeared to arrange an assortment of hormonal systems, administrative proteins, and different qualities, keeping cells alive and solid.

Their past work has uncovered that in the mind, sirt1 ensures against the neurodegeneration seen in Alzheimer's, Huntington's and Parkinson's ailments.

"Sirt1 is a protein that expels acetyl bunches from different proteins, changing their movement. The potential focuses of this deacetylation are various, which is likely what gives sirt1 its wide scope of defensive forces," Guarente says.

In the cell metabolism study, the specialists investigated the several qualities that were turned on in mice lacking sirt1 yet encouraged a typical eating regimen and found that they were practically indistinguishable from those turned on in ordinary mice sustained a high-fat eating regimen.

This recommends in typical mice, improvement of the metabolic issue is a two-advance procedure. "the initial step is inactivation of sirt1 by the high-fat eating routine, and the subsequent advance is all the terrible things that follow that," Guarente says. The scientists explored how this happens and found that in ordinary mice given a high-fat eating routine, the sirt1 protein is cut by a compound called caspase-1, which is instigated by irritation. It's now realized that high-fat eating regimens can incite irritation; however, it's hazy precisely how that occurs, Guarente says. "what our examination says is that once you incite the fiery reaction, the outcome in the fat cells is that sirt1 WILL be severed," he says.

That discovering "gives a pleasant sub-atomic system to see how fiery signals in fat tissue could prompt quick unhinging of metabolic tissue," says Anthony Suave, a partner teacher of pharmacology at Weill Cornell medical college, who was not part of the exploration group.

Medications that focus on that incendiary procedure, just as medications that improve sirtuin action, may have some gainful remedial impact against heftiness related issues, suave says.

Chapter 4: How do sirtfoods and the diet work?

The basis of the sirtuin diet can be explained in simple terms or in complex ways. It is important to understand how and why it works, however, so that you can appreciate the value of what you are doing. It is important to also know why these sirtuin rich foods help to help you maintain fidelity to your diet plan. Otherwise, you may throw something in your meal with less nutrition that would defeat the purpose of planning for one rich in sirtuins. Most importantly, this is not a dietary fad, and as you will see, there is much wisdom contained in how humans have used natural foods even for medicinal purposes, over thousands of years.

To understand how the sirtfood diet works, and why these particular foods are necessary, we will look at the role they play in the human body.

Sirtuin activity was first researched in yeast, where a mutation caused an extension in the yeast's lifespan. Sirtuins were also shown to slow ageing in laboratory mice, fruit flies, and nematodes. As research on sirtuins proved to transfer to mammals, they were examined for their use in diet and slowing the ageing process. The sirtuins in humans are different in type, but they essentially work in the same ways and reasons.

There are seven "members" that make up the sirtuin family. It is believed that sirtuins play a big role in regulating certain functions of cells, including proliferation (reproduction and growth of cells), apoptosis (death of cells). They promote survival and resist stress to increase longevity.

They are also seen to block neurodegeneration (loss of function of the nerve cells in the brain). They conduct their housekeeping functions by cleaning out toxic proteins and supporting the brain's ability to change and adapt to different conditions, or to recuperate (i.e., brain plasticity). As part of this, they also help reduce chronic inflammation and reduce something called oxidative stress. Oxidative stress is when there are too many cell-damaging free radicals circulating in the body, and the body cannot catch up by combating them with anti-oxidants. These factors are related to age-related illness and weight as well, which again, brings us back to a discussion of how they actually work.

You will see labels in sirtuins that start with "sir," which represents "silence information regulator" genes. They do exactly that, silence or regulate, as part of their functions. The seven sirtuins that humans work with are: sirt1, sirt2, sirt3, sirt4, sirt 5, sirt6 and sirt7. Each of these types is responsible for different areas of protecting cells. They work by either stimulating or turning on certain gene expressions, or by reducing and turning off other gene expressions. This essentially means that they can influence genes to do more or less of something, most of which they are already programmed to do.

Through enzyme reactions, each of the sirt types affects different areas of cells that are responsible for the metabolic processes that help to maintain life. This is also related to what organs and functions they will affect.

For example, the sirt6 causes an expression of genes in humans that affect skeletal muscle, fat tissue, brain, and heart. Sirt 3 would cause an expression of genes that affect the kidneys, liver, brain and heart.

If we tie these concepts together, you can see that the sirtuin proteins can change the expression of genes, and in the case of the sirtfood diet, we care about how sirtuins can turn off those genes that are responsible for speeding up ageing and for weight management.

The other aspect to this conversation of sirtuins is the function and the power of calorie restriction on the human body. Calorie restriction is simply eating fewer calories. This, coupled with exercise and reducing stress, is usually a combination of weight loss. Calorie restriction has also proven across much research in animals and humans to increase one's lifespan.

We can look further at the role of sirtuins with calorie restriction, and using the sirt3 protein, which has a role in metabolism and ageing. Amongst all of the effects of the protein on gene expression, (such as preventing cells from dying, reducing tumours from growing, etc.), we want to understand the effects of sirt3 on weight for the purpose of this book.

The sirt3 has high expression in those metabolically active tissues as we stated earlier, and its ability to express itself increases with caloric restriction, fasting, and exercise. On the contrary, it will express itself less when the body has a high fat, high-calorie-riddleddiet.

The last few highlights of sirtuins are their role in regulating telomeres and reducing inflammation which also helps with staving off disease and ageing.

Telomeres are sequences of proteins at the ends of chromosomes. When cells divide, these get shorter. As we age, they get shorter, and other stressors to the body also will contribute to this. Maintaining these longer telomeres is the key to slower ageing. In addition, proper diet, along with exercise and other variables, can lengthen telomeres. Sirt6 is one of the sirtuins that, if activated, can help with DNA damage, inflammation and oxidative stress. Sirt1 also helps with inflammatory response cycles that are related to many age-related diseases.

Calories restriction, as we mentioned earlier, can extend life to some degree.

Since this, as well as fasting, is a stressor, these factors will stimulate the sirt3 proteins to kick in and protect the body from the stressors and excess free radicals. Again, the telomere length is affected as well.

Having laid this all out before you, you should be able to appreciate how and why these miraculous compounds work in your favour, to keep you youthful, healthy, and lean if they are working hard for you, don't you feel that you should do something too? Well, you can, and that is what the rest of this book will do for you.

Getting started on sirtfoods

So, after you have just filled your head with more molecular biology information that you probably needed to since high school or college, let us look at next steps of how to proceed with the sirtfood diet, and also how to fill your refrigerator.

Starting the sirtfood diet is very easy. It just takes a bit of preparation. If you do not know what kale is, or where you would find green tea, then you may have a learning curve, albeit very small. There is little in the way of starting the sirtfood diet.

Since you will be preparing and cooking healthy foods, you may want to do a few things the week you start:

1. Clear your cabinets and refrigerator of foods that are obviously unhealthy, and that might tempt you. You also will have a very low-calorie intake at the start, and you do not want to be tempted into a quick fix that may set you back. Even though you will have new recipes, you may feel that your old comfort foods are easier at the moment.

2. Go shopping for all of the ingredients that you will need for the week. If you buy what you will need, it is more cost-effective. Also, once you see the recipes, you will notice that there are many ingredients that overlap. You will get to know your portions as you proceed with the diet, but at least you will have what you need and save yourself some trips to the store.

3. Wash, dry, cut and store all of the foods that you need that way you have them conveniently prepared when you need them. This will make a new diet seem less tedious.

One necessary kitchen tool that you will need aside from the actual foods is a juicer. You will need a juicer as soon as you start the sirtfood diet. Juicers are everywhere, so they are quite easy to find, but the quality ranges greatly, however. This is where price, function, and convenience comes into play. You could go to a popular department store, or you can find them online. Once you know what you are going after, you can shop around.

Here are some other tips to help you get started:

Drink your juices as the earlier meals in the day if it helps you. It is a great way to start your day for three reasons.

- it will give you energy for breakfast and for lunch, especially. By not having to digest heavy foods, your body saves time and energy usually spent on moving things around to go through all the laborious motions. You will be guaranteed to feel lighter and more energetic this way. You can always change this pattern after the maintenance phase, but you may find that you want to keep that schedule.
- having fruits and vegetables before starchy or cooked meals, no matter how healthy the ingredients are the best way to go for your digestion. Fruits and vegetables digest more rapidly, and the breakdown into the compounds that we can use more readily. Think of it as having your salad before your dinner. It works in the same way. The heavier foods, grains, oils, meats, etc., take more time to digest. If you eat these first, they will slow things

down, and that is where you have a backup of food needing to be broken down. This is also when you may find yourself with indigestion.

- juices, especially green juices, contain phytochemicals that not only serve as anti-oxidants, but they contribute to our energy and mood. You will notice that you feel much differently after drinking a green juice than you would if you had eggs and sausage. You may want to make a food diary and note things such as this!

Be prepared to adjust to having lighter breakfasts for a little while. Most often, we fill up with high protein, carbohydrate, and high-calorie meals early in the day. We may feel that we did not get enough to eat and that we are not full at first. Oddly as it sounds, we may even miss the action of chewing. Some people need to chew their food to feel like they have had a filling meal. It is something automatic that we do not think of. Some also will miss that crunch such as with toast. Just pay attention to this, and know this is normal, and that it will pass.

Sirtfoods for all

Numerous wellbeing cognizant individuals are focused on a specific style of eating, with any semblance of discontinuous fasting with the 5:2 and different weight control plans, low-carb, including the Dukan diet, paleo and without gluten eats less being particularly mainstream while they don't work for a few, many vouches for them.

Be that as it may, how do sirtfoods fit in with these different weight control plans?

1. sirtfoods are good with all other dietary **Directions:**ologies as well as can effectively improve their advantages.
2. Low-carb counts calories that need plant-based nourishments can be drastically enlarged by the consideration of sirtfoods.
3. sirtfoods are the regular paleo nourishments, containing the sirtuin-enacting polyphenols that people would have developed eating and receiving the rewards from over an exceptionally extensive stretch of time.
4. The best 20 sirtfoods are normally without gluten making them a genuine advantage for anybody following a sans gluten diet.

Masters of muscle

The rising incidence of corpulence related ailments, for example, diabetes, dyslipidemia, and cardiovascular and cerebrovascular sicknesses in industrialized nations have become a general medical issue vital. Numerous helpful and preventive systems to forestall or battle corpulence have come around; however, few have endured the trial of time. One marvel that got the enthusiasm for this setting is the alleged "French oddity." first noted by Irish doctor Samuel Black in 1819, the French catch 22 makes an inference to the way that the French are seen as having a moderately low occurrence of cardiovascular and metabolic infection, despite the fact that their eating regimen is wealthy in immersed fat. The high utilization of red wine, which is rich in the polyphenol resveratrol, is believed to be one of the essential elements adding to this particular preferred position.

In the interim, since the 1930s, it has been likewise notable that caloric limitation (cr) can hinder the maturing procedure and defer the beginning of various maturing related illnesses, for example, malignancy, cardiovascular infections, and metabolic ailments. Cr altogether extends life expectancy in living beings running from yeast and nematodes to rodents and monkeys (1, 2). Strikingly, the valuable wellbeing results of cr look like those that are prompted by resveratrol in various creature models, proposing that the atomic pathways by which resveratrol acts are like those initiated by cr.

As of late, it was proposed that the sirtuins could be the regular go-betweens that clarify both the impacts of resveratrol and cr pathways. In this survey, we will talk about the atomic system that underlies the organic action of these sirtuins, their useful jobs in entire body physiology, and their potential relationship to human maladies.

Chapter 5: Top twenty sirtfoods

These are the best 20 sirtfoods and the establishment of the sirtfood diet.

- • sirtuins are ace metabolic controllers that control our capacity to consume fat and remain solid
- • sirtuins go about as vitality sensors inside our cells and are initiated when a deficiency of vitality is recognized
- fasting and exercise both initiate our sirtuin qualities yet these can be difficult to continue on with and may have disadvantages

By eating an eating regimen wealthy in the main 20 sirtfoods, you can copy the impacts of fasting and practise and accomplish a more advantageous body.

Buckwheat	**Other sirtfoods**
Capers	
Celery	*Fruits:*
Chicory (red)	
Chilli (bird's eye variety)	Apples
Cocoa	Blackberries
Coffee	Blackcurrants
Green tea	Blueberries
Kale	Cranberries
Medjool dates	Fruits
olives & olive oil	Goji berries
Onion (red)	Grapes (red)
Parsley	Kumquats
Red wine	Plums
Rocket (arugula)	Raspberries
Soy & tofu products	
Strawberries	*Vegetables:*
Turmeric (ground)	
Walnuts	Artichokes
	Asparagus
	Broad beans
	Broccoli

Cannellini beans

Chestnuts

chia seeds

Chicory (yellow)

Chilli peppers

Chives

Corn (popcorn)

Dill

Endive lettuce

Ginger

Green beans

Haricot beans

Onions (white)

Oregano

Pak choi (bok choy)

Peanuts

Peppermint

Pistachios

Quinoa

Sage

Shallots

sunflower seeds

Watercress

Wholemeal flour

Chapter 6: Cancer preventing superfoods

The heart of this diet is, of course, the food selection. Sirtuin activators are all found in plants, but you have to take note that not all veggies and fruits have the necessary compound to consider it as sirtfood. Examples of this non-sirtuin activator food are avocados (very popular in the world of losing weight), cucumber, bananas and carrots, although it doesn't mean that these type of fruits and veggies are not packed with benefits or not worth eating. But for our purpose, which is to tap on our body's sirtuin, you have to make sure that you will follow the list (and research more) and include it in your daily diet.

Aside from promoting fat burning and muscle gain, most sirtfood is also full of other nutritional benefits. Here are some of the top sirtuin-activator food selections: *green tea (preferable matcha powder)* - a better alternative than your builder's tea is green tea. Green tea is made from steamed fresh leaves from the plant instead of the fermented leaves. This sirtuin-filled beverage is actually a popular choice for health buffs, making it the world's most consumed beverage after water. It is known to help boost weight loss, prevent Alzheimer's disease, reduce cholesterol build-up, and combat heart diseases. Some of the essential vitamins and minerals it contains are folate, vitamin b, magnesium and other antioxidants.

Dark chocolate - not just any kind of chocolate (but equally satisfying and has lower fat and sugar content), your choice should have at least 85% cocoa solids in order to be considered as sirtfood.

Kale - this is a popular "superfood" since it is filled with antioxidants (beta-carotene, kaempferol, quercetin and more). In fact, this veggie has one of the highest oxygen radical absorbance capacity or orac rating; it is known to be nutrient-dense – it has omega 3 fatty acids, vitamins a, k,C and b6, it also has calcium, potassium, magnesium and more. It can also lower cholesterol levels, has anti-cancer effects and can help you lose weight.

Parsley - adding this popular herb to your meal is very easy as sprinkling it on your steak and other delicious dishes. This sirtuin food has vitamins a,C and k (richest herbal source for vitamin k). This sirtuin-rich food also contains volatile oil and flavonoid. It is also said to help promote osteotropic activity in our bones.

olives and extra-virgin olive oil - olive oil is one of the mainstays of the Mediterranean diet for a good reason. olives and extra-virgin olive oil can help reduce cholesterol, contains dietary fibre, and is also rich in essential vitamins and minerals such as iron, potassium, magnesium, iodine, phosphorus and more.

Onions (red onion is the maximum sirtuin activator) - aside from adding flavour to our dishes, onion is actually a popular component for different home remedies. It is known to heal infection, reduce inflammation and regulates sugar. In addition, it also has high polyphenol content, contains volatile oil and other organic sulfur compounds.

Turmeric – curcumin, a substance found in turmeric, has potent anti-inflammatory effects. Aside from being a strong antioxidant, it is also known for its anti-inflammatory effects. It is also known to help with liver problems, arthritis, heartburn, kidney problems, and even depression. Other suggest that turmeric should be used in conjunction with black pepper for a better effect.

Blackcurrants - this is another powerhouse of antioxidants, especially with anthocyanins. This berry has a high level of vitamin c. It is known to help fight diabetes, heart failure and reduce risk of stroke and heart attack.

Blueberries - the perfect add on for your breakfast oats, or cereals are also rich in vitamin c, k and fibre.

Strawberries - another one from the berry family, this one is also rich in anthocyanins like blackcurrants. This compound is said to aid in reducing high blood pressure.

Apples - most likely, you have heard the saying, "an apple a day, keeps the doctor away," and indeed, apples are really | Servings: your health. Aside from being a sirtuin activator, it is also known to help lower cholesterol levels and has a good amount of fibre, which can help put those hunger pangs away as it can make you feel fuller and satiated.

Omega-3 fish oil - usually found in fish and is known to lower blood pressure, reduce abnormal heart rhythm and the likelihood of a heart attack. This supplement can ward off heart-related diseases.

Capers - these little buds are rich in flavonoid compounds quercetin and rutin, which can strengthen the capillaries (small blood vessels). It also has healthy levels of vitamins k, a, riboflavin and niacin.

Passion fruit - a good source of phytochemical piceatannol (choose fresh and not canned).

Tofu - this soy-based food is a good source of isoflavones, which is known to help boost sirtuins. Experts suggest that tofu should be consumed along with onions, asparagus and garlic (these 3 can help the body absorb the isoflavones).

Red wine (preferably pinot noir) - this drink contains resveratrol, which is known to trigger sirtuins. Red wine is often pointed to as one of the main reasons for the French's slim figure; it is also rich in antioxidants and is known to benefit the heart.

Other sirtuin-rich foods include chillies, celery, coffee, lovage, buckwheat, Medjool dates, walnuts, citrus fruits, chicory (choose red) and rocket. You can also further research on plant-based foods under sirtfood for more choices and alternatives.

There are a lot of ways to include these type of foods in your diet. You can also experiment and research different dishes so that you can add in these ingredients.

Chapter 7: Breakfast

Sirt food cocktail

Preparation time: 5 minutes | Cooking time: 0 minutes | Servings: 4

Ingredients:

75g (3oz) kale

50g (2oz) strawberries

1 apple, cored

2 sticks of celery

1 tbsp parsley

1 tsp of matcha powder

Squeeze lemon juice (optional) to taste

Directions:

Place the ingredients into a blender and add enough water to cover the ingredients and blitz to a smooth consistency.

Summer berry smoothie

Preparation time: 5 minutes | Cooking time: 0 minutes | Servings: 4

Ingredients:

50g (2oz) blueberries

50g (2oz) strawberries

25G (1oz) blackcurrants

25G (1oz) red grapes

1 carrot, peeled

1 orange, peeled

Juice of 1 lime

Directions:

Place all of the ingredients into a blender and cover them with water.

Blitz until smooth.

You can also add some crushed ice and a mint leaf to garnish.

Mango, celery & ginger smoothie

Preparation time: 10 minutes | Cooking time: 0 minutes | Servings: 4

Ingredients:

1 stalk of celery

50g (2oz) kale

1 apple, cored

50g (2oz) mango, peeled, de-stoned and chopped

2.5cm (1-inch) chunk of fresh ginger root, peeled and chopped

Directions:

Put all the ingredients into a blender with some water and blitz until smooth.

Add ice to make your smoothie really refreshing.

Orange, carrot & kale smoothie

Preparation time: 5 minutes | Cooking time: 0 minutes | Servings: 4

Ingredients:

1 carrot, peeled

1 orange, peeled

1 stick of celery

1 apple, cored

50g (2oz) kale

½ tsp matcha powder

Directions:

Place all of the ingredients into a blender and add in enough water to cover them.

Process until smooth, serve and enjoy.

Creamy strawberry & cherry smoothie

Preparation time: 5 minutes | Cooking time: 0 minutes | Servings: 4

Ingredients:

100g (3½ oz) strawberries

75g (3oz) frozen pitted cherries

1 tbsp plain full-fat yoghurt

175ML (6fl oz) unsweetened soya milk

Directions:

Place all of the ingredients into a blender and process until smooth.

Serve and enjoy.

Grape, celery & parsley reviver

Preparation time: 5 minutes | Cooking time: 0 minutes | Servings: 4

Ingredients:

75g (3oz) red grapes

3 sticks of celery

1 avocado, de-stoned and peeled

1 tbsp fresh parsley

½ tsp matcha powder

Directions:

Place all of the ingredients into a blender with enough water to cover them and blitz until smooth and creamy.

Add crushed ice to make it even more refreshing.

Strawberry & citrus blend

Preparation time: 5 minutes | Cooking time: 0 minutes | Servings: 4

Ingredients:

75g (3oz) strawberries

1 apple, cored

1 orange, peeled

½ avocado, peeled and de-stoned

½ tsp matcha powder

Juice of 1 lime

Directions:

Place all of the ingredients into a blender with enough water to cover them and process until smooth.

Sirtfood mushroom scrambled eggs

Preparation time: 5 minutes | Cooking time: 40 minutes | Servings: 3

Ingredients:

2 eggs

1 tsp ground turmeric

1 tsp gentle curry powder

20g kale, generally hacked

1 tsp additional virgin olive oil

½ 10,000Foot bean stew, daintily cut

Bunch of catch mushrooms, daintily cut

5g parsley, finely slashed

optional add a seed blend as a topper and some rooster sauce for enhance

Directions:

Blend the turmeric and curry powder and include a little water until you have accomplished a light glue.

Steam the kale for 2-3 minutes.

Warmth the oil in a griddle over medium heat and fry the stew and mushrooms for 2-3 minutes until they have begun to dark coloured and soften.

Grapefruit & celery blast

Preparation time: 5 minutes | Cooking time: 0 minutes | Servings: 4

Ingredients:

1 grapefruit, peeled

2 stalks of celery

50g (20z) kale

½ tsp matcha powder

Directions:

Place all the ingredients into a blender with enough water to cover them and blitz until smooth.

Orange & celery crush

Preparation time: 5 minutes | Cooking time: 0 minutes | Servings: 4

Ingredients:

1 carrot, peeled

3 stalks of celery

1 orange, peeled

½ tsp matcha powder

Juice of 1 lime

Directions:

Place all of the ingredients into a blender with enough water to cover them and blitz until smooth.

Tropical chocolate delight

Preparation time: 5 minutes | Cooking time: 0 minutes | Servings: 4

Ingredients:

1 mango, peeled & de-stoned

75g (3oz) fresh pineapple, chopped

50g (20z) kale

25G (10Z) rocket

1 tbsp 100% cocoa powder or cacao nibs

150Ml (5fl oz) coconut milk

Directions:

Place all of the ingredients into a blender and blitz until smooth.

You can add a little water if it seems too thick.

Walnut & spiced apple tonic

Preparation time: 5 minutes | Cooking time: 0 minutes | Servings: 4

Ingredients:

6 walnuts halves

1 apple, cored

1 banana

½ tsp matcha powder

½ tsp cinnamon

Pinch of ground nutmeg

Directions:

Place all of the ingredients into a blender and add sufficient water to cover them.

Blitz until smooth and creamy.

Pineapple & cucumber smoothie

Preparation time: 5 minutes | Cooking time: 0 minutes | Servings: 4

Ingredients:

50g (2oz) cucumber

1 stalk of celery

2 slices of fresh pineapple

2 sprigs of parsley

½ tsp matcha powder

Squeeze of lemon juice

Directions:

Place all of the ingredients into a blender with enough water to cover them and blitz until smooth.

Sweet rocket (arugula) boost

Preparation time: 5 minutes | Cooking time: 0 minutes | Servings: 4

Ingredients:

25G (1OZ) fresh rocket (arugula) leaves

75g (3oz) kale

1 apple

1 carrot

1 tbsp fresh parsley

Juice of 1 lime

Directions:

Place all of the ingredients into a blender with enough water to cover and process until smooth.

Avocado, celery & pineapple smoothie

Preparation time: 5 minutes | Cooking time: 0 minutes | Servings: 4

Ingredients:

50g (2oz) fresh pineapple, peeled and chopped

3 stalks of celery

1 avocado, peeled & de-stoned

1 tsp fresh parsley

½ tsp matcha powder

Juice of ½ lemon

Directions:

Place all of the ingredients into a blender and add enough water to cover them.

Process until creamy and smooth.

Banana & ginger snap

Preparation time: 5 minutes | Cooking time: 0 minutes | Servings: 4

Ingredients:

2.5cm (1-inch) chunk of fresh ginger, peeled

1 banana

1 large carrot

1 apple, cored

½ stick of celery

¼ level tsp turmeric powder

Directions:

Place all the ingredients into a blender with just enough water to cover them.

Process until smooth.

Chocolate, strawberry & coconut crush

Preparation time: 5 minutes | Cooking time: 0 minutes | Servings: 4

Ingredients:

100ml (3½fl oz) coconut milk

100g (3½oz) strawberries

1 banana

1 tbsp 100% cocoa powder or cacao nibs

1 tsp matcha powder

Directions:

Toss all of the ingredients into a blender and process them to a creamy consistency.

Add a little extra water if you need to thin it a little.

Chocolate berry blend

Preparation time: 5 minutes | Cooking time: 0 minutes | Servings: 4

Ingredients:

50g (2oz) kale

50g (2oz) blueberries

50g (2oz) strawberries

1 banana

1 tbsp 100% cocoa powder or cacao nibs

200ml (7fl oz) unsweetened soya milk

Directions:

Place all of the ingredients into a blender with enough water to cover them and process until smooth.

Cranberry & kale crush

Preparation time: 5 minutes | Cooking time: 0 minutes | Servings: 4

Ingredients:

75g (3oz) strawberries

50g (2oz) kale

120ml (4fl oz) unsweetened cranberry juice

1 tsp chia seeds

½ tsp matcha powder

| Servings: 1

71 calories per serving

Directions:

Place all of the ingredients into a blender and process until smooth.

Add some crushed ice and a mint leaf or two for a really refreshing drink.

Poached eggs & rocket (arugula)

Preparation time: 5 minutes | Cooking time: 10 minutes | Servings: 4

Ingredients:

2 eggs

25G (1OZ) fresh rocket (arugula)

1 tsp olive oil

sea salt

freshly ground black pepper

Directions:

Scatter the rocket (arugula) leaves onto a plate and drizzle the olive oil over them.

Bring a shallow pan of water to the boil, add in the eggs and cook until the whites become firm.

Serve the eggs on top of the rocket and season with salt and pepper.

Strawberry buckwheat pancakes

Preparation time: 5 minutes | Cooking time: 25 minutes | Servings: 4

Ingredients:

100g (3½oz) strawberries, chopped

100g (3½ oz) buckwheat flour

1 egg

250ML (8fl oz) milk

1 tsp olive oil

1 tsp olive oil for frying

freshly squeezed juice of 1 orange

Directions:

Pour the milk into a bowl and mix in the egg and a tsp of olive oil.

Sift in the flour to the liquid mixture until smooth and creamy.

Allow it to rest for 15 minutes.

Heat a little oil in a pan and pour in a quarter of the mixture (or to the size you prefer.)

Sprinkle in a quarter of the strawberries into the batter.

Cook for around 2 minutes on each side.

Serve hot with a drizzle of orange juice.

You could try experimenting with other berries such as blueberries and blackberries.

Strawberry & nut granola

Preparation time: 5 minutes | Cooking time: 25 minutes | Servings: 4

Ingredients:

200g (7oz) oats

250G (9oz) buckwheat flakes

100g (3½ oz) walnuts, chopped

100g (3½ oz) almonds, chopped

100g (3½ oz) dried strawberries

1½ tsp ground ginger

1½ tsp ground cinnamon

120ml (4fl oz) olive oil

2 tbsp honey

Directions:

Combine the oats, buckwheat flakes, nuts, ginger and cinnamon.

In a saucepan, warm the oil and honey.

Stir until the honey has melted.

Pour the warm oil into the dry ingredients and mix well.

Spread the mixture out on a large baking tray (or two) and bake in the oven at 150C (300F) for around 50 minutes until the granola is golden.

Allow it to cool.

Add in the dried berries.

Store in an airtight container until ready to use.

Can be served with yoghurt, milk or even dry as a handy snack.

Chilled strawberry & walnut porridge

Preparation time: 5 minutes | Cooking time: 20 minutes | Servings: 4

Ingredients:

100g (3½ oz) strawberries

50g (2oz) rolled oats

4 walnut halves, chopped

1 tsp chia seeds

200ml (7fl oz) unsweetened soya milk

100ml (3½ fl oz) water

Directions:

Place the strawberries, oats, soya milk and water into a blender and process until smooth.

Stir in the chia seeds and mix well.

Chill in the fridge overnight and serve in the morning with a sprinkling of chopped walnuts.

It's simple and delicious.

Fruit & nut yoghurt crunch

Preparation time: 5 minutes | Cooking time: 25 minutes | Servings: 4

Ingredients:

100g (3½ oz) plain Greek yoghurt

50g (2oz) strawberries, chopped

6 walnut halves, chopped

Sprinkling of cocoa powder

Directions:

Stir half of the chopped strawberries into the yoghurt.

Using a glass, place a layer of yoghurt with a sprinkling of strawberries and walnuts, followed by another layer of the same until you reach the top of the glass.

Garnish with walnuts pieces and a dusting of cocoa powder.

Cheesy baked eggs

Preparation time: 5 minutes | Cooking time: 25 minutes | Servings: 4

Ingredients:

4 large eggs

75g (3oz) cheese, grated

25G (1OZ) fresh rocket (arugula) leaves, finely chopped

1 tbsp parsley

½ tsp ground turmeric

1 tbsp olive oil

Directions:

Grease each ramekin dish with a little olive oil.

Divide the rocket (arugula) between the ramekin dishes then break an egg intoeach one.

Sprinkle a little parsley and turmeric on top then sprinkle on the cheese.

Place the ramekins in a preheated oven at 220C/425F for 15 minutes, until the eggs are set, and the cheese is bubbling.

Green egg scrambled

Preparation time: 5 minutes | Cooking time: 30 minutes | Servings: 4

Ingredients:

2 eggs, whisked

25G (1OZ) rocket (arugula) leaves

1 tsp chives, chopped

1 tsp fresh basil, chopped

1 tsp fresh parsley, chopped

1 tbsp olive oil

Directions:

Mix the eggs together with the rocket (arugula) and herbs.

Heat the oil in a frying pan and pour into the egg mixture.

Gently stir until it's lightly scrambled.

Season and serve.

Spiced scrambled

Preparation time: 5 minutes | Cooking time: 25 minutes | Servings: 4

Ingredients:

25G (1OZ) kale, finely chopped

2 eggs

1 spring onion (scallion) finely chopped

1 tsp turmeric

1 tbsp olive oil

sea salt

freshly ground black pepper

Directions:

Crack the eggs into a bowl.

Add the turmeric and whisk them.

Season with salt and pepper.

Heat the oil in a frying pan, add the kale and spring onions (scallions) and cook until it has wilted.

Pour in the beaten eggs and stir until eggs have scrambled together with the kale.

olive, tomato & herb frittata

Preparation time: 5 minutes | Cooking time: 25 minutes | Servings: 4

Ingredients:

50g (2oz) cheddar cheese, grated (shredded)

75g (3oz) pitted black olives, halved

8 cherry tomatoes, halved

4 large eggs

1 tbsp fresh parsley, chopped

1 tsp fresh basil, chopped

1 tbsp olive oil

Directions:

Break the eggs into a bowl and whisk them then add in the parsley, basil, olives and tomatoes.

Add in the cheese and stir it.

Heat the oil in a small frying pan and pour in the egg mixture.

Cook until the egg mixture completely sets.

Place the frittata under a hot grill for 3 minutes to finish it off.

Carefully remove it from the pan.

Cut into slices and serve.

Mushroom & red onion buckwheat pancakes

Preparation time: 5 minutes | Cooking time: 35 minutes | Servings: 4

Ingredients:

For the pancakes 125g (4oz) buckwheat flour 1 egg

150ml (5fl oz) semi-skimmed milk

150ml (5fl oz) water

1 tsp olive oil for frying for the filling

1 red onion, chopped

75g (3½ oz) mushrooms, sliced

50g (2oz) spinach leaves

1 tbsp fresh parsley, chopped

1 tsp olive oil

50g (2oz) rocket (arugula) leaves

Directions:

Sift the flour into a bowl and mix in an egg. Pour in the milk and water and mix to a smooth batter.

Set aside.

Heat a tsp of olive oil in a pan.

Add the onion and mushrooms and cook for 5 minutes.

Add the spinach and allow it to wilt.

Set aside and keep it warm.

Heat a tsp of oil in a frying pan and pour in half of the batter.

Cook for 2 minutes on each side until golden.

Spoon the spinach and mushroom mixture onto the pancake and add the parsley.

Fold it over and serve onto a scattering of rocket (arugula) leaves.

Repeat for the remaining mixture.

Kale & feta salad with cranberry dressing

Preparation time: 5 minutes | Cooking time: 30 minutes | Servings: 4

Ingredients:

250G (9oz) kale, finely chopped

50g (2oz) walnuts, chopped

75g (3oz) feta cheese, crumbled

1 apple, peeled, cored and sliced

4 Medjool dates, chopped

For the dressing:

75g (3oz) cranberries

½ red onion, chopped

3 tbsp olive oil

3 tbsp water

2 tsp honey

1 tbsp red wine vinegar sea salt

Directions:

Place the ingredients for the dressing into a food processor and process until smooth.

If it seems too thick, you can add a little extra water if necessary.

Place all the ingredients for the salad into a bowl.

Pour on the dressing and toss the salad until it is well coated in the mixture.

Tuna, egg & caper salad

Preparation time: 5 minutes | Cooking time: 35 minutes | Servings: 4

Ingredients:

100g (3½oz) red chicory (or yellow if not available)

150G (5oz) tinned tuna flakes in brine, drained

100g (3 ½ oz) cucumber

25G (1oz) rocket (arugula)

6 pitted black olives

2 hard-boiled eggs, peeled andquartered

2 tomatoes, chopped

2 tbsp fresh parsley, chopped

1 red onion, chopped

1 stalk of celery

1 tbsp capers

2 tbsp garlic vinaigrette (see recipe)

Directions:

Place the tuna, cucumber, olives, tomatoes, onion, chicory, celery, parsley and rocket (arugula) into a bowl.

Pour in the vinaigrette and toss the salad in the dressing.

Serve onto plates and scatter the eggs and capers on top.

Hot chicory & nut salad

Preparation time: 5 minutes | Cooking time: 25 minutes | Servings: 4

Ingredients:

For the salad:

100g (3½oz) green beans

100g (3½oz) red chicory, chopped (if unavailable use yellow chicory)

100g (3½oz) celery, chopped

25G (1OZ) macadamia nuts, chopped

25G (1OZ) walnuts, chopped

25G (1OZ) plain peanuts, chopped

2 tomatoes, chopped

1 tbsp olive oil

For the dressing:

2 tbsp fresh parsley, finely chopped

½ tsp turmeric

½ tsp mustard

1 tbsp olive oil

25ML (1Fl oz) red wine vinegar

Directions:

Mix together the ingredients for the dressing then set them aside.

Heat a tbsp of olive oil in a frying pan then add the green beans, chicory and celery.

Cook until the vegetables have softened then add in the chopped tomatoes and cook for 2 minutes.

Add the prepared dressing, and thoroughly coat all of the vegetables.

Serve onto plates and sprinkle the mixture of nuts over the top.

Eat immediately.

Honey chilli squash

Peparation time: 5 minutes | Cooking time: 40 minutes | Servings: 4

Ingredients:

2 red onions, roughly chopped

2.5cm (1-inch) chunk of ginger root, finely chopped

2 cloves of garlic

2 bird's eye chillies, finely chopped

1 butternut squash, peeled and chopped

100ml (3½ fl oz) vegetable stock (broth)

1 tbsp olive oil

Juice of 1 orange

Juice of 1 lime

2 tsp honey

Directions:

Warm the oil into a pan and add in the red onions, squash chunks, chillies, garlic, ginger and honey.

Cook for 3 minutes.

Squeeze in the lime and orange juice.

Pour in the stock (broth), orange and lime juice and cook for 15 minutes until tender.

Serrano ham & rocket (arugula)

Preparation time: 5 minutes | Cooking time: 25 minutes | Servings: 4

Ingredients:

175G (6oz) serrano ham

125g (4oz) rocket (arugula) leaves

2 tbsp olive oil

1 tbsp orange juice

Directions:

Pour the oil and juice into a bowl and toss the rocket (arugula) in the mixture.

Serve the rocket onto plates and top it off with the ham.

Buckwheat pasta salad

Preparation time: 5 minutes | Cooking time: 35 minutes | Servings: 4

Ingredients:

275G (10oz) buckwheat pasta

225g (8oz) green beans

100g (3½ oz) cherry tomatoes

2 cloves of garlic, crushed

1 red onion, finely chopped

1 bird's eye chilli, finely chopped

2 tbsp smooth peanut butter

150Ml (5fl oz) coconut milk

1 tbsp tomato puree

½ tsp turmeric powder

2 tbsp olive oil.

Directions:

Cook the buckwheat according to the directions, then set aside and keep warm.

Heat the olive oil in a large frying pan or wok.

Add the garlic and onion and cook for 1 minute.

Add in the green beans and cook for 3 minutes.

Add in the tomatoes and cook for 2 minutes.

In a separate bowl mix the peanut butter, coconut milk, turmeric, tomato puree and chilli.

Add the pasta and coconut mixture to the vegetables.

Stir well, making sure everything is well coated.

Serve alongside a leafy green salad.

Hot chorizo, tomato & kale salad

Preparation time: 5 minutes | Cooking time: 20 minutes | Servings: 4

Ingredients:

225g (8oz) kale leaves, finely chopped

75g (3oz) chorizo sausage, thinly sliced

8 cherry tomatoes

2 cloves of garlic

1 red onion, finely chopped

2 tbsp olive oil

2 tbsp red wine vinegar sea salt

freshly ground black pepper

Directions:

Heat the olive oil into a frying pan and add the sliced chorizo, garlic, onion and tomatoes.

Cook for around 5 minutes.

Add in the red wine vinegar and kale and cook for around 7 minutes or until the kale has softened.

Season with salt and pepper.

Serve immediately.

Red chicory & walnut coleslaw

Preparation time: 5 minutes | Cooking time: 45 minutes | Servings: 4

Ingredients:

100g (3½ oz) red chicory, (or yellow) finely grated (shredded)

5 stalks of celery, finely chopped

8 walnut halves, chopped

1 red onion, finely chopped

2 tbsp mayonnaise

Directions:

Place all of the ingredients into a bowl and combine well.

Chill in the fridge before serving.

Smoked salmon & chicory boats

Preparation time: 5 minutes | Cooking time: 25 minutes | Servings: 4

Ingredients:

150G (5oz) red chicory leaves (or yellow if it's unavailable)

150G (5oz) smoked salmon, finely chopped

100g (3½oz) cucumber, diced

2 tbsp fresh parsley, chopped

½ red onion, finely chopped

Juice of 1 lime

2 tbsp olive oil

Directions:

Place the salmon, cucumber, onion, parsley, oil and lime juice into a bowl and toss the ingredients well.

Scoop some of the salmon mixtures into each of the chicory leaves and chill before serving.

Vegetable & nut loaf

Preparation time: 5 minutes | Cooking time: 35 minutes | Servings: 4

Ingredients:

175G (6oz) mushrooms, finely chopped

100g (3½ oz) haricot beans

100g (3½ oz) walnuts, finely chopped

100g (3½ oz) peanuts, finely chopped

1 carrot, finely chopped

3 sticks celery, finely chopped

1 bird's eye chilli, finely chopped

1 red onion, finely chopped

1 egg, beaten

2 cloves of garlic, chopped

2 tbsp olive oil

2 tsp turmeric powder

2 tbsp soy sauce

4 tbsp fresh parsley, chopped

100ml (3½ fl oz) water

60ml (2Fl oz) red wine

Directions:

Heat the oil in a pan and add the garlic, chilli, carrot, celery, onion, mushrooms and turmeric.

Cook for 5 minutes.

Place the haricot beans in a bowl and stir in the nuts, vegetables, soy sauce, egg, parsley, red wine and water.

Grease and line a large loaf tin with greaseproof paper.

Spoon the mixture into the loaf tin, cover with foil and bake in the oven at 190C/375F for 60-90 minutes.

Let it stand for 10 minutes then turn onto a serving plate.

Dates & parma ham

Preparation time: 5 minutes | Cooking time: 25 minutes | Servings: 4

Ingredients:

12 Medjool dates

2 slices of parma ham, cut into strips

Directions:

Wrap each date with a strip of parma ham.

Can be served hot or cold.

Braised celery

Preparation time: 5 minutes | Cooking time: 15 minutes | Servings: 4

Ingredients:

250G (9oz) celery, chopped

100ml (3½ fl oz) warm vegetable stock (broth)

1 red onion, chopped

1 clove of garlic, crushed

1 tbsp fresh parsley, chopped

25G (1oz) butter

sea salt and freshly ground black pepper

Directions:

Place the celery, onion, stock (broth) and garlic into a saucepan and bring it to the boil, reduce the heat and simmer for 10 minutes.

Stir in the parsley and butter and season with salt and pepper.

Serve as an accompaniment to roast meat dishes.

Cheesy buckwheat cakes

Preparation time: 5 minutes | Cooking time: 30 minutes | Servings: 4

Ingredients:

100g (3½oz) buckwheat, cooked and cooled

1 large egg

25G (1oz) cheddar cheese, grated (shredded)

25G (1oz) wholemeal breadcrumbs

2 shallots, chopped

2 tbsp fresh parsley, chopped

1 tbsp olive oil

Directions:

Crack the egg into a bowl, whisk it then set aside.

In a separate bowl combine all the buckwheat, cheese, shallots and parsley and mix well.

Pour in the beaten egg to the buckwheat mixture and stir well.

Shape the mixture into patties.

Scatter the breadcrumbs on a plate and roll the patties in them.

Heat the olive oil in a large frying pan and gently place the cakes in the oil.

Cook for 3-4 minutes on either side until slightly golden.

Red chicory & stilton cheese boats

Preparation time: 5 minutes | Cooking time: 25 minutes | Servings: 4

Ingredients:

200g (7oz) stilton cheese, crumbled

200g (7oz) red chicory leaves (or if unavailable, use yellow)

2 tbsp fresh parsley, chopped 1 tbsp olive oil

Directions:

Place the red chicory leaves onto a baking sheet.

Drizzle them with olive oil then sprinkle the cheese inside the leaves.

Place them under a hot grill (broiler) for around 4 minutes until the cheese has melted.

Sprinkle with chopped parsley and serve straight away.

Strawberry, rocket (arugula) & feta salad

Preparation time: 5 minutes | Cooking time: 50 minutes | Servings: 4

Ingredients:

75g (3oz) fresh rocket (arugula) leaves

75g (3oz) feta cheese, crumbled

100g (3½ oz) strawberries, halved

8 walnut halves

2 tbsp flaxseeds

Directions:

Combine all the ingredients in a bowl then scatter them onto two plates.

For an extra sirtfood boost you can drizzle over some olive oil.

Mushroom courgetti & lemon caper pesto

Preparation time: 5 minutes | Cooking time: 25 minutes | Servings: 4

Ingredients:

4 courgettes (zucchinis)

10 oyster mushrooms, sliced

1 red onion, sliced

2 tbsp olive oil

2 tbsp lemon caper pesto (see recipe)

50g (2oz) rocket (arugula) leaves

Directions:

Spiralize the courgettes into spaghetti.

If you don't have a spiralizer, finely cut the vegetables lengthways into long 'spaghetti' strips.

Heat the olive oil in a frying pan, add the mushrooms and onions and cook for minutes.

Add in the courgettes and the pesto and cook for 5 minutes.

Scatter the rocket (arugula) leaves onto plates and serve the courgettes on top.

Chicken stir-fry

Preparation time: 5 minutes | Cooking time: 20 minutes | Servings: 4

Ingredients:

150G (5oz) egg noodles

50g (2oz) cauliflower florets, roughly chopped

25G (1oz) kale, finely chopped

25G (1oz) mange tout

2 sticks of celery, finely chopped

2 chicken breasts

1 red pepper (bell pepper),chopped

1 clove of garlic

2 tbsp soy sauce

100ml (3½ fl oz) chicken stock (broth)

1 tbsp olive oil

Directions:

Cook the noodles according to the directions, then set aside and keep warm.

Heat the oil in a wok or frying pan and add in the garlic and chicken.

Add in the kale, celery, cauliflower, red pepper (bell pepper), mange tout and cook for 4 minutes.

Pour in the chicken stock (broth) and soy sauce and cook for 3 minutes or until the chicken is thoroughly cooked.

Stir in the cooked noodles and serve.

Tuna with lemon herb dressing

Preparation time: 5 minutes | Cooking time: 15 minutes | Servings: 4

Ingredients:

4 tuna steaks

1 tbsp olive oil

For the dressing:

25G (1oz) pitted green olives, chopped

2 tbsp fresh parsley, chopped

1 tbsp fresh basil, chopped

2 tbsp olive oil

freshly squeezed juice of 1 lemon

Directions:

Heat a tbsp of olive oil in a griddle pan.

Add the tuna steaks and cook on high heat for 2-3 minutes on each side.

Reduce the cooking time if you want them rare.

Place the ingredients for the dressing into a bowl and combine them well.

Serve the tuna steaks with a dollop of dressing over them.

Serve alongside a leafy rocket salad.

Kale, apple & fennel soup

Preparation time: 5 minutes | Cooking time: 20 minutes | Servings: 4

Ingredients:

450g (1Lb) kale, chopped

200g (7oz) fennel, chopped

2 apples, peeled, cored and chopped

2 tbsp fresh parsley, chopped

1 tbsp olive oil

sea salt

freshly ground black pepper

Directions:

Heat the oil in a saucepan, add the kale and fennel and cook for 5 minutes until the fennel has softened.

Stir in the apples and parsley.

Cover with hot water, bring it to the boil and simmer for 10 minutes.

Using a hand blender or food processor blitz until the soup is smooth.

Season with salt and pepper.

Lentil soup

Preparation time: 5 minutes | Cooking time: 25 minutes | Servings: 4

Ingredients:

175G (6oz) red lentils

1 red onion, chopped

1 clove of garlic, chopped

2 sticks of celery, chopped

2 carrots, chopped

½ bird's eye chilli

1 tsp ground cumin

1 tsp ground turmeric

1 tsp ground coriander (cilantro)

1200ml (2 pints) vegetable stock (broth)

2 tbsp olive oil

salt and pepper

Directions:

Heat the oil in a saucepan and add the onion and cook for 5 minutes.

Add in the carrots, lentils, celery, chilli, coriander (cilantro), cumin, turmeric and garlic and cook for 5 minutes.

Pour in the stock (broth), bring it to the boil, reduce the heat and simmer for 45 minutes.

Using a hand blender or food processor, puree the soup until smooth.

Season with salt and pepper.

Serve.

Cauliflower & walnut soup

Preparation time: 5 minutes | Cooking time: 15 minutes | Servings: 4

Ingredients:

450g (1Lb) cauliflower, chopped

8 walnut halves, chopped

1 red onion, chopped

900ml (1½ pints) vegetable stock (broth)

100ml (3½ fl oz) double cream (heavy cream)

½ tsp turmeric

1 tbsp olive oil

Directions:

Heat the oil in a saucepan, add the cauliflower and red onion and cook for 4 minutes, stirring continuously.

Pour in the stock (broth), bring to the boil and cook for 15 minutes.

Stir in the walnuts, double cream and turmeric.

Using a food processor or hand blender, process the soup until smooth and creamy.

Serve into bowls and top off with a sprinkling of chopped walnuts.

Celery & blue cheese soup

Preparation time: 5 minutes | Cooking time: 25 minutes | Servings: 4

Ingredients:

125g (4oz) blue cheese

25G (1OZ) butter

1 head of celery (approx 65 0g)

1 red onion, chopped

900ml (1½ pints) chicken stock (broth)

150Ml (5fl oz) single cream

Directions:

Heat the butter in a saucepan, add the onion and celery and cook until the vegetables have softened.

Pour in the stock, bring to the boil then reduce the heat and simmer for 15 minutes.

Pour in the cream and stir in the cheese until it has melted.

Serve and eat straight away.

Spicy squash soup

Preparation time: 5 minutes | Cooking time: 35 minutes | | Servings: 4

Ingredients:

150G (5oz) kale

1 butternut squash, peeled, de-seeded and chopped

1 red onion, chopped

3 bird's eye chillies, chopped

3 cloves of garlic

2 tsp turmeric

1 tsp ground ginger

600ml (1 pint) vegetable stock (broth)

2 tbsp olive oil

Directions:

Heat the olive oil in a saucepan, add the chopped butternut squash and onion and cook for 6 minutes until softened.

Stir in the kale, garlic, chilli, turmeric and ginger and cook for 2 minutes, stirring constantly.

Pour in the vegetable stock (broth) bring it to the boil and cook for 20 minutes.

Using a food processor or a hand blender process until smooth.

Serve on its own or with a swirl of cream or Crème Fraiche.

Enjoy.

French onion soup

Preparation time: 5 minutes | Cooking time: 25 minutes | Servings: 4

Ingredients:

750g (1¾Lbs) red onions, thinly sliced

50g (2oz) cheddar cheese, grated (shredded)

12G (½ oz) butter

2 tsp flour

2 slices wholemeal bread

900ml (1½ pints) beef stock (broth)

1 tbsp olive oil

Directions:

Heat the butter and oil in a large pan.

Add the onions and gently cook on low heat for 25 minutes, stirring occasionally.

Add in the flour and stir well. Pour in the stock (broth) and keep stirring.

Bring to the boil, reduce the heat and simmer for 30 minutes.

Cut the slices of bread into triangles, sprinkle with cheese and place them under a hot grill (broiler) until the cheese has melted.

Serve the soup into bowls and add 2 triangles of cheesy toast on top and enjoy.

Cream of broccoli & kale soup

Preparation time: 5 minutes | Cooking time: 35 minutes | Servings: 4

Ingredients:

250G (9oz) broccoli

250G (9oz) kale

1 potato, peeled and chopped

1 red onion, chopped

600ml (1 pint) vegetable stock

300ml (½ pint) milk

1 tbsp olive oil

sea salt

freshly ground black pepper

Directions:

Heat the olive oil in a saucepan, add the onion and cook for 5 minutes.

Add in the potato, kale and broccoli and cook for 5 minutes.

Pour in the stock (broth) and milk and simmer for 20 minutes.

Using a food processor or hand blender, process the soup until smooth and creamy.

Season with salt and pepper.

Re-heat if necessary and serve.

Chapter 8: Salads

Arugula salad with Italian dressing

Preparation time: 5 minutes | Cooking time: 0 minutes | Servings: 4

Ingredients:

2 cups of arugula

1 cup of shredded cabbage

Italian dressing

Cayenne pepper (optional)

Few sprigs of parsley

2 tbsp chopped red onions

Strawberry arugula salad

Preparation time: 5 minutes | Cooking time: 0 minutes | Servings: 4

Ingredients:

2 tbsp black sesame seeds

1 tbsp poppy seeds

½ cup olive oil

¼ cup lemon juice

¼ tsp paprika

1 bag fresh arugula - chopped, washed and dried

1-quart strawberries, sliced

Directions:

Whisk together the sesame seeds, olive oil, poppy seeds, paprika, lemon juice and onion. Refrigerate.

In a large bowl, combine arugula, strawberries and walnuts.

Pour dressing over salad.

Toss and refrigerate 15 minutes before serving.

Kale, grilled shrimp & eggs salad

Preparation time: 5 minutes | Cooking time: 0 minutes | Servings: 4

Ingredients:

1½ cup grilled shrimp

1 cup chopped kale leaves

3 hard-boiled quartered eggs

Dressing:

1 tbsp olive oil or avocado oil

1 tbsp fresh lemon juice

Pinch of black pepper

Pinch of sea salt

Directions:

mix all ingredients.

Kale, almond & avocado salad

Preparation time: 5 minutes | Cooking time: 0 minutes | Servings: 4

Ingredients:

1½ cup chopped kale

½ cup almonds

2 chopped avocado

Dressing:

1 tbsp olive oil or avocado oil

1 tbsp fresh lemon juice

Pinch of black pepper

Pinch of sea salt

Directions:

Mix all ingredients.

Kale, melon, & tomato salad

Preparation time: 5 minutes | Cooking time: 0 minutes | Servings: 4

Ingredients:

2 cup cubed melon

1 cup chopped kale

2 cup cherry tomatoes

1 cup lettuce

Dressing:

1 tbsp olive oil or avocado oil

1 tbsp fresh lemon juice

Pinch of black pepper

Pinch of sea salt

Directions:

Mix all ingredients.

Kale, grapefruit, toasted almonds & parmesan salad

Preparation time: 5 minutes | Cooking time: 0 minutes | Servings: 4

Ingredients:

½ cup toasted almonds

½ cup parmesan shavings

2 red grapefruits, flesh only, skins removed

2 cups kale, chopped and massaged with olive oil and salt

Dressing:

1 tbsp olive oil or avocado oil

1 tbsp fresh lemon juice

Pinch of black pepper

Pinch of sea salt

Directions:

Mix all ingredients.

Kale, walnut & pomegranate salad

Preparation time: 5 minutes | Cooking time: 0 minutes | Servings: 4

Ingredients: 1 cup walnuts

1 cup pomegranate seeds

2 cups kale, chopped and massaged with olive oil and salt

Dressing:

1 tbsp olive oil or avocado oil

1 tbsp fresh lemon juice

Pinch of black peppe

Pinch of sea salt

Directions: Mix all ingredients.

Pork & kale salad

Preparation time: 5 minutes | Cooking time: 20 minutes | Servings: 4

Ingredients:

1Lb pork roast

2 cups steamed kale

Dressing:

1 tbsp olive oil or avocado oil

1 tbsp fresh lemon juice

Pinch of black pepper

Pinch of sea salt

Directions:

Steam kale, season and place pork roast on top of kale.

Slice pork roast and let roast juices mingle with kale for few minutes.

Mediterranean spinach salad

Preparation time: 5 minutes | Cooking time: 0 minutes | Servings: 3

Ingredients:

1 bag baby spinach, washed and dried

4-5 spring onions, finely chopped

1 cucumber, peeled and cut

½ cup walnuts, halved and roasted

1/3 cup yoghurt

2 tbsp red wine vinegar

3 tbsp extra virgin olive oil

salt and black pepper, to taste

Directions:

Whisk yoghurt, olive oil and vinegar in a small bowl.

Place the baby spinach leaves in a large salad bowl.

Add the onions, cucumber and walnuts.

Season with black pepper and salt, stir and toss with the dressing.

Summer green bean salad

Preparation time: 5 minutes | Cooking time: 10 minutes | Servings: 4

Ingredients:

1Lb trimmed green beans, cut to 2-3-inch long pieces

1 small red onion, finely cut

1 cup cherry tomatoes, halved

1 avocado, peeled, pitted and cut

3-4 garlic cloves, chopped

1 tbsp chia seeds

4 tbsp extra virgin olive oil

¾ cup freshly grated parmesan cheese

salt and pepper, to taste

1 cup fresh dill, finely cut, to serve

Directions:

Steam or boil the green beans for about 3-4 minutes until crisp-tender.

In a colander, wash with cold water to stop cooking, then pat dry and place in a salad bowl.

Add red onion, garlic, cherry tomatoes, and avocado and sprinkle in the chia seeds.

Season with lemon juice and balsamic vinegar.

Toss to coat, add in the olive oil and parmesan cheese and toss again.

Season to taste with salt and freshly ground black pepper.

Refrigerate for an hour and serve sprinkled with fresh dill.

Warm beet and lentil salad

Preparation time: 5 minutes | Cooking time: 0 minutes

Ingredients:

1 14 oz can brown lentils, drained, rinsed

1 14 oz can sliced pickled beets, drained

1 cup baby arugula leaves

1 small red onion, chopped

2 garlic cloves, crushed

6 oz feta cheese, crumbled

1 tbsp extra virgin olive oil

For the dressing:

3 tbsp extra virgin olive oil

1 tbsp red wine vinegar

1 tsp summer savoury

salt and black pepper, to taste

Directions:

Heat one tbsp of olive oil in a frying pan and gently sauté onion for 2-3 minutes or until softened.

Add in garlic, lentils and beets.

Cook, stirring, for 2 minutes.

Whisk together remaining olive oil, vinegar, summer savoury, salt andpepper.

Add to the lentils and toss to coat.

Combine baby arugula, feta and lentil mixture in a bowl.

Toss gently to combine and serve.

Roasted vegetable salad

Preparation time: 5 minutes | Cooking time: 20 minutes | Servings: 4-5

Ingredients:

3 tomatoes, halved

1 zucchini, quartered

1 fennel bulb, thinly sliced

2 small eggplants, ends trimmed, quartered

1 large red pepper, halved, deseeded, cut into strips

2 medium onions, quartered

1 tsp oregano

2 tbsp extra virgin olive oil

For the dressing:

2/3 cup yoghurt

1 tbsp fresh lemon juice

1 small garlic clove, chopped

Directions:

Place the zucchini, eggplant, pepper, fennel, onions, tomatoes and olive oil on a lined baking sheet.

Season with salt, pepper and oregano and roast in a 500F oven until golden, about 20 minutes.

Whisk the yoghurt, lemon juice and garlic in a bowl.

Taste and season with salt and pepper.

Divide the vegetables onto 4-5 plates.

Top with the yoghurt mixture and serve.

Warm leek and sweet potato salad

Preparation time: 5 minutes | Cooking time: 30 minutes | Servings: 4-5

Ingredients:

1.5lb sweet potato, unpeeled, cut into 1-inch pieces

4 small leeks, trimmed and cut into 1-inch slices

5-6 white mushrooms, halved

1 cup baby arugula leaves

2 tbsp extra virgin olive oil

For the dressing:

½ cup yoghurt

1 tbsp dijon mustard

Directions:

Preheat oven to 350F.

Line a baking tray with baking paper.

Place the sweet potato, leeks and mushrooms on the baking tray.

Drizzle with olive oil and toss to coat.

Roast for 20 minutes or until golden.

Combine yoghurt and mustard in a small bowl or cup.

Place vegetables, mushrooms and baby arugula in a salad bowl and toss to combine.

Serve drizzled with the yoghurt mixture.

Warm tomato salad

Preparation time: 5 minutes | Cooking time: 10 minutes | Servings: 4-5

Ingredients:

4 tomatoes, sliced

1 cup cherry tomatoes, halved

½ small red onion, very finely cut

2 garlic cloves, crushed

1 tbsp dried mint

2 tbsp extra virgin olive oil

1 tbsp balsamic vinegar

Directions:

Gently heat oil in a nonstick frying pan over low heat.

Cook garlic and tomatoes, occasionally stirring, for 4-5

minutes or until tomatoes are warm but firm.

Remove from heat and place in a plate.

Add in red onion, vinegar and dried mint.

Season with salt and pepper to taste and serve.

Shredded kale and brussels sprout salad

Preparation time: 10 minutes | Cooking time: 20 minutes | Servings: 4-6

Ingredients:

18-29 brussels sprouts, shredded

1 cup finely shredded kale

½ cup grated parmesan or pecorino cheese

1 cup walnuts, halved, toasted

½ cup dried cranberries

For the dressing:

6 tbsp extra virgin olive oil

2 tbsp apple cider vinegar

1 tbsp dijon mustard

salt and pepper, to taste

Directions:

Shred the brussels sprouts and kale in a food processor or mandolin.

Toss them in a bowl, top with toasted walnuts, cranberries and grated cheese.

In a smaller bowl, whisk the olive oil, apple cider vinegar and mustard until smooth.

Pour the dressing over the salad, stir and serve.

Quinoa and zucchini ribbon salad

Preparation time: 10 minutes | Cooking time: 40 minutes | Servings: 4

Ingredients:

1 cup quinoa

2 cups of water

1 zucchini, sliced lengthways into thin ribbons (a mandoline is ideal)

3-4 green onions, chopped

1 cup cherry tomatoes, halved

4 oz feta, crumbled or cut in small cubes

2 tbsp extra virgin olive oil

3 tbsp lemon juice

salt, to taste

Directions:

Heat oil in a large saucepan over medium-high heat.

Add zucchini and cook, stirring, until zucchini is crisp-tender, about 4 minutes.

Set aside in a plate.

Wash quinoa in a fine-mesh strainer under running water for 1-2 minutes, then set aside to drain.

Bring water to a boil in a medium saucepan over high heat.

Add in the quinoa and return to a boil.

Cover, reduce heat to a simmer and cook gently for 15 minutes.

Set aside, covered, for 5-6 minutes.

Toss quinoa with zucchini, green onions, tomatoes, lemon juice and olive oil.

Serve warm or room temperature, topped with feta cheese.

Quinoa and avocado salad

Preparation time: 10 minutes | Cooking time: 20 minutes | Servings: 4

Ingredients:

1 cup quinoa 2 cups of water

1 large avocado, pitted and sliced

¼ radicchio, finely sliced

1 small pink grapefruit, peeled and finely cut

1 handful arugula

1 cup baby spinach leaves

2 tbsp extra virgin olive oil

2 tbsp lemon juice

salt and black pepper, to taste

Directions:

Wash quinoa in a fine sieve under running water for 2-3 minutes, or until water runs clear.

Set aside to drain, then boil it in two cups of water for 15 minutes.

Fluff with a fork and set aside to cool.

Stir avocado, radicchio, arugula and baby spinach into cooled quinoa.

Add grapefruit, lemon juice, and olive oil, season with salt and black pepper and stir to combine well.

Quinoa and carrot salad

Preparation time: 10 minutes | Cooking time: 0 minutes | Servings: 4

Ingredients: 1 cup quinoa

2 cups of water 4 carrots, shredded

1 apple, peeled and shredded

1 garlic clove, chopped

3 tbsp lemon juice

2 tbsp extra virgin olive oil

salt, to taste

Directions:

Rinse the quinoa very well in a sieve under running water and set aside to drain.

Boil two cups of water, add in the quinoa and simmer for 15 minutes.

Fluff with a fork and set aside to cool.

In a deep salad bowl, combine the shredded carrots, apple and lemon juice, garlic and salt.

Add in the cooled quinoa, toss to combine and serve.

Quinoa, kale and roasted pumpkin

Preparation time: 10 minutes | Cooking time: 20 minutes | Servings: 4-5

Ingredients: 1 cup quinoa

2 cups of water

1.5Lb pumpkin, peeled and seeded, cut into cubes

2 cups fresh kale, chopped

5 oz crumbled feta cheese

1 large onion, finely chopped

4-5 tbsp extra virgin olive oil

1 tsp finely grated ginger ½ tsp cumin

½ tsp salt

Directions: Preheat oven to 350F.

Line a baking tray and arrange the pumpkin cubes on it.

Drizzle with 2-3 tbsp of olive oil and salt.

Toss to coat, place in the oven and cook for 20-25 minutes, stirring every 10 minutes.

Heat the remaining olive oil in a large saucepan over medium-high heat.

Gently sauté onion, for 2-3 minutes, or until softened. Add the spices and cook, stirring, for 1 minute more.

Wash quinoa under running water until the water runs clear. Bring two cups of water to a boil and add quinoa. Reduce heat to low, cover, and simmer for 15 minutes.

Stir in kale and cook until it wilts.

Gently combine quinoa and kale mixture with the roasted pumpkin and sautéed onion.

Buckwheat salad with broccoli and roasted peppers

Preparation time: 10 minutes | Cooking time: 10 minutes | Servings: 4

Ingredients:

1 cup buckwheat groats

1 ¾ cups vegetable broth

1 small broccoli head, cut into florets

2-3 roasted bell peppers, peeled and cut

1 red onion, finely chopped

3 garlic cloves, crushed or chopped

1 tbsp balsamic vinegar

2-3 tbsp extra virgin olive oil

½ cup fresh dill, finely cut, to serve salt and black pepper, to taste

Directions:

Toast the buckwheat in a dry saucepan for about 2 minutes, stirring.

Bring the vegetable broth to a boil and add it gently to the buckwheat.

Reduce heat, cover, and simmer for 5 minutes, or until the buckwheat is tender.

Remove from heat and fluff with a fork.

Arrange broccoli on a baking sheet and drizzle with garlic, olive oil, balsamic vinegar and salt.

Toss to coat.

Roast in a preheated to 350F oven for about 20 minutes, or until tender.

Transfer the broccoli in a large salad bowl along with the roasted peppers and buckwheat.

Stir in red onion.

Sprinkle with dill and toss gently.

Warm mushroom buckwheat salad

Preparation time: 10 minutes | Cooking time: 20 minutes | Servings: 4

Ingredients: 1 cup buckwheat groats

1 ¾ cups vegetable broth

5-6 green onions, chopped

10-12 white mushrooms, sliced

1 tbsp dried thyme

1 cup sun-dried tomatoes, cut

2 tbsp extra virgin olive oil salt, to taste

Black pepper, optional

Directions: Toast the buckwheat in a dry saucepan for about 2 minutes, stirring.

Boil the vegetable broth and add it gently to the buckwheat. Reduce heat, cover, and simmer for 5 minutes, or until the buckwheat is tender. Remove from heat and fluff with a fork. Heat olive oil in a frying pan and gently sauté the green onions for 1-2 minutes.

Stir in mushrooms, thyme, and season with salt, to taste.

Cook, stirring until the mushrooms soften and most of the liquid evaporates.

Combine the warm buckwheat with the mushrooms and dried tomatoes and serve.

Easy chickpea salad

Preparation time: 10 minutes | Cooking time: 10 minutes | Servings: 3-4

Ingredients:

1 15 oz can of chickpeas, drained

1 medium red onion, finely cut

1 cucumber, peeled and diced

2 tomatoes, sliced

A bunch of radishes, sliced

½ cup fresh parsley, finely chopped

2 tbsp extra virgin olive oil

1 tbsp balsamic vinegar salt, to taste

4 oz crumbled feta cheese, to serve

Directions:

In a salad bowl, toss together the chickpeas, onion, cucumber, tomatoes, radishes and parsley.

Add in the balsamic vinegar, olive oil and salt and stir.

Serve sprinkled with crumbled feta cheese.

Chapter 9: Desserts and snacks

Superfoods raw vegan cookies

Preparation time: 10 minutes | Cooking time: 30 minutes | Servings: 4

Ingredients:

½ cup of coconut milk

½ cup of cocoa powder

½ cup of coconut oil

½ cup raw honey

2 cups finely shredded coconut

1 cup large flake coconut

2 tsp of ground vanilla bean

½ cup chopped almonds or chia seeds (optional)

½ cup almond butter (optional)

Directions:

Combine the coconut milk, cocoa powder and coconut oil in a saucepan.

I think that it still counts as a raw dessert if you have to warm up the coconut milk and coconut oil.

So, warm up the mixture over medium heat because we want the coconut oil to melt and become liquid.

Raw vegan walnuts pie crust & raw brownies

Preparation time: 10 minutes | Cooking time: 30 minutes | Servings: 4

Ingredients:

1½ cups walnuts

1 cup pitted dates

1½ tsp ground vanilla bean

2 tsp chia seeds

1/3 cup unsweetened cocoa powder

Topping for raw brownies:

1/3 cup almond butter

Directions:

Add walnuts to a food processor or blender.

Mix until finely ground.

Add the vanilla, dates, and cocoa powder to the blender.

Mix well and optionally add a couple of drops of water at a time to make the mixture stick together.

This is a basic raw walnuts pie crust recipe.

You can use almonds or cashews as well.

If you need a pie crust, then spread it thinly in a 9-inch disc and add the filling.

If you want to make raw brownies, then transfer the mixture into a small dish and top with almond butter.

Raw vegan Reese's cups

Preparation time: 10 minutes | Cooking time: 35 minutes | Servings: 4

Ingredients:

 "Peanut" butter filling

½ cup sunflower seeds butter

½ cup almond butter

1 tbsp raw honey

2 tbsp melted coconut oil

Superfoods chocolate part:

½ cup cacao powder

2 tbsp raw honey

1/3 cup of coconut oil (melted)

Directions:

Mix the "peanut" butter filling ingredients.

Put a spoonful of the mixture into each muffin cup.

Refrigerate.

Mix superfoods chocolate ingredients.

Put a spoonful of the superfoods chocolate mixture over the "peanut" butter mixture. Freeze!

Raw vegan coffee cashew cream cake

Preparation time: 10 minutes | Cooking time: 35 minutes | Servings: 4

Ingredients:

Coffee cashew cream

2 cups raw cashews

1 tsp of ground vanilla bean

3 tbsp melted coconut oil

¼ cup raw honey

1/3 cup very strong coffee or triple espresso shot

For the crust:

See recipe for *Raw Walnuts Pie Crust*

Directions:

Blend all ingredients for the cream, pour it onto the crust and refrigerate.

Garnish with coffee beans.

Raw vegan chocolate cashew truffles

Preparation time: 10 minutes | Cooking time: 35 minutes | Servings: 4

Ingredients:

1 cup ground cashews

1 tsp of ground vanilla bean

½ cup of coconut oil

¼ cup raw honey

2 tbsp flax meal

2 tbsp hemp hearts

2 tbsp cacao powder

Directions:

Mix all ingredients and make truffles. Sprinkle coconut flakes on top.

Raw vegan double almond raw chocolate tart

Preparation time: 10 minutes | Cooking time: 35 minutes | Servings: 4

Ingredients:

1½ cups of raw almonds

¼ cup of coconut oil, melted

1 tbsp raw honey or royal jelly

8 ounces dark chocolate, chopped

1 cup of coconut milk

½ cup unsweetened shredded coconut

Directions:

Crust:

Ground almonds and add melted coconut oil, raw honey and combine.

Using a spatula, spread this mixture into the tart or pie pan.

Filling:

Put the chopped chocolate in a bowl, heat coconut milk and pour over chocolate and whisk together.

Pour filling into tart shell.

Refrigerate.

Toast almond slivers chips and sprinkle over tart.

Raw vegan bounty bars

Preparation time: 10 minutes | Cooking time: 35 minutes | Servings: 4

Ingredients:

"Peanut" butter filling

2 cups desiccated coconut

3 tbsp coconut oil - melted

1 cup of coconut cream - full fat

4 tbsp of raw honey

1 tsp ground vanilla bean

Pinch of sea salt

Superfoods chocolate part:

½ cup cacao powder

2 tbsp raw honey

1/3 cup of coconut oil (melted)

Directions:

Mix coconut oil, coconut cream, honey, vanilla and salt.

Pour over desiccated coconut and mix well.

Mould coconut mixture into balls, small bars similar to bounty and freeze.

Or pour the whole mixture into a tray, freeze and cut into small bars.

Make superfoods chocolate mixture, warm it up and dip frozen coconut into the chocolate and put on a tray and freeze again.

Raw vegan tartlets with coconut cream

Preparation time: 10 minutes | Cooking time: 35 minutes | Servings: 4

Ingredients:

Crust:

See recipe for *Raw Walnuts Pie Crust*.

Make tartlets.

Pudding:

1 avocado

2 tbsp coconut oil

2 tbsp raw honey

2 tbsp cacao powder

1 tsp ground vanilla bean

Pinch of salt

¼ cup almond milk, as needed

Coconut cream:

See recipe for *Whipped Coconut Cream.*

Add ½ tsp cinnamon and whip again.

To make the pudding:

Blend all the ingredients in the food processor until smooth and thick.

Spread evenly into tartlet crusts.

Optionally, put some goji berries on top of the pudding layer.

Make the coconut cream, spread it on top of the pudding layer, and put back in the fridge overnight.

Serve with one blueberry on top of each tartlet.

Raw vegan "peanut" butter truffles

Preparation time: 10 minutes | Cooking time: 30 minutes | Servings: 4

Ingredients:

5 tbsp sunflower seed butter

1 tbsp coconut oil

1 tbsp raw honey

1 tsp ground vanilla bean

¾ cup almond flour

1 tbsp flaxseed meal

Pinch of salt

1 tbsp cacao butter

hemp hearts (optional)

¼ cup superfoods chocolate

Directions:

Mix until all ingredients are incorporated.

Roll the dough into 1-inch balls, place them on parchment paper and refrigerate for half an hour (yield about 14 truffles).

Dip each truffle in the melted superfoods chocolate, one at the time.

Place them back on the pan with parchment paper or coat them in cocoa powder or coconut flakes.

Raw vegan chocolate pie

Preparation time: 10 minutes | Cooking time: 25 minutes | Servings: 4

Ingredients:

Crust:

2 cups almonds, soaked overnight and drained

1 cup pitted dates, soaked overnight and drained

1 cup chopped dried apricots

1½ tsp ground vanilla bean

2 tsp chia seeds

1 banana

Filling:

4 tbsp raw cacao powder

3 tbsp raw honey

2 ripe avocados

2 tbsp organic coconut oil

2 tbsp almond milk (if needed, check for consistency first)

Directions:

Add almonds and banana to a food processor or blender.

Mix until it forms a thick ball.

Add the vanilla, dates, and apricot chunks to the blender.

Mix well and optionally add a couple of drops of water at a time to make the mixture stick together.

Spread in a 10-inch dis.

Mix filling ingredients in a blender andadd almond milk if necessary.

Add filling to the crust and refrigerate.

Raw vegan chocolate walnut truffles

Preparation time: 10 minutes | Cooking time: 35 minutes | Servings: 4

Ingredients:

1 cup ground walnuts

1 tsp cinnamon

½ cup of coconut oil

¼ cup raw honey

2 tbsp chia seeds

2 tbsp cacao powder

Directions:

Mix all ingredients and make truffles.

Coat with cinnamon, coconut flakes or chopped almonds.

Raw vegan carrot cake

Preparation time: 10 minutes | Cooking time: 35 minutes | Servings: 4

Ingredients:

Crust:

4 carrots, chopped

1½ cups oats

½ cup dried coconut

2 cups dates

1 tsp cinnamon

½ tsp nutmeg

1½ cups cashews

2 tbsp coconut oil

Juice from 1 lemon

2 tbsp raw honey

1 tsp ground vanilla bean

Water, as needed

Directions:

Add all crust ingredients to the blender.

Mix well and optionally add a couple of drops of water at a time to make the mixture stick together.

Press in a small pan.

Take it out and put on a plate and freeze.

Mix frosting ingredients in a blender and add water if necessary.

Add frosting to the crust and refrigerate.

Frozen raw blackberry cake

Preparation time: 10 minutes | Cooking time: 45 minutes | Servings: 4

Ingredients:

Crust:

¾ cup shredded coconut

15 dried dates soaked in hot water and drained

1/3 cup pumpkin seeds

¼ cup of coconut oil

Middle filling

Coconut whipped cream - see *Coconut Whipped Cream* recipes.

Top filling:

1 pound of frozen blackberries

3-4 tbsp raw honey

¼ cup of coconut cream

2 egg whites

Directions:

Grease the cake tin with coconut oil and mix all base ingredients in the blender until you get a sticky ball.

Press the base mixture in a cake tin.

Freeze.

Make *Coconut Whipped Cream*.

Process berries and add honey, coconut cream and egg whites.

Pour middle filling - *Coconut Whipped Cream* in the tin and spread evenly.

Freeze.

Pour top filling - berries mixture-in the tin, spread, decorate with blueberries and almonds and return to freezer.

Raw vegan chocolate hazelnuts truffles

Preparation time: 10 minutes | Cooking time: 30 minutes | Servings: 4

Ingredients:

1 cup ground almonds

1 tsp ground vanilla bean

½ cup of coconut oil

½ cup mashed pitted dates

12 whole hazelnuts

2 tbsp cacao powder

Directions:

Mix all ingredients and make truffles with one whole hazelnut in the middle.

Raw vegan chocolate cream fruity cake

Preparation time: 10 minutes | Cooking time: 45 minutes | Servings: 4

Ingredients:

Crust:

See *Raw Walnut Pie Crust* recipe

Chocolate cream:

1 avocado

2 tbsp raw honey

2 tbsp coconut oil

2 tbsp cacao powder

1 tsp ground vanilla bean

Pinch of sea salt

¼ cup of coconut milk

1 tbsp coconut flakes

Fruits:

1 chopped banana

1 cup pitted cherries

Top layer:

Coconut whipped cream - see *Coconut Whipped Cream* recipes.

Directions:

Prepare the crust and press it at the bottom of the pan.

Blend all chocolate cream ingredients, fold in the fruits and pour in the crust.

Whip the top layer, spread and sprinkle with cacao powder.

Refrigerate.

Raw vegan carob sesame truffles

Preparation time: 10 minutes | Cooking time: 35 minutes | Servings: 4

Ingredients:

1 cup ground walnuts

1 tsp ground vanilla bean

½ cup of coconut oil

½ cup mashed pitted dates

3 tbsp *carob powder*

3 tbsp chia seeds

Directions:

Mix all ingredients and make truffles.

Coat with slivered almond or sesame seeds.

Raw vegan almond date cherry pie

Preparation time: 10 minutes | Cooking time: 35 minutes | Servings: 4

Ingredients:

Crust:

2 cups almonds, soaked overnight and drained

1 cup pitted dates, soaked overnight and drained

1½ tsp ground vanilla bean

1 tsp cinnamon powder

A pinch of nutmeg

1 banana

Middle layer:

1 cup pitted cherries

Filling:

4 tbsp raw cacao powder

3 tbsp raw honey

2 ripe avocados

2 tbsp organic coconut oil

2 tbsp almond milk (if needed, check for consistency first)

Directions:

Mix crust ingredients and spread in a 10-inch disk.

Mix filling ingredients in a blender and add almond milk if necessary.

Spread cherries on the crust, pour filling over, sprinkle with coconut flakes and refrigerate.

Raw vegan seeds truffles

Preparation time: 10 minutes | Cooking time: 25 minutes | Servings: 4

Ingredients:

½ cup ground sunflower seeds

½ cup ground pumpkin seeds

1 tbsp chia seeds

1 tbsp Sesame seeds

1 tsp cinnamon

½ cup of coconut oil

½ cup mashed pitted dates

3 tbsp cacao powder

Directions:

Mix all ingredients and make truffles.

Coat with cocoa powder, coconut flakes or ground pumpkin seeds.

Vegan apple spice cookies

Preparation time: 10 minutes | Cooking time: 35 minutes | Servings: 4

Ingredients:

1 cup unsweetened almond butter

½ cup raw honey

1 egg

½ tsp salt

1 apple, diced

1 tsp cinnamon

¼ tsp ground cloves

1/8 tsp nutmeg

1 tsp fresh ginger, grated

Directions:

Heat oven to 350F.

Combine almond butter, egg, raw honey and salt in a bowl.

Add apple, spices, and ginger and stir.

Spoon batter onto a baking sheet 1-inches apart.

Bake until set.

Remove cookies and allow to cool on a cooling rack.

Superfoods macaroons

Preparation time: 10 minutes | Cooking time: 30 minutes | Servings: 4

Ingredients:

3 egg whites

½ cup of coconut sugar

¼ tsp salt

1 cup unsweetened flaked coconut

½ cup soft dried apricots, coarsely chopped (3 ounces)

Directions:

Heat the oven to 325F.

Whisk together egg whites, sugar, and salt in a bowl until frothy.

Add apricots and coconut and mix to combine.

Shape mixture into mounds with hands and place one-inch apart on the baking sheet.

Bake until lightly golden, 35-40 minutes.

Rotate sheet halfway through.

You can cover them with superfoods dark chocolate.

Pumpkin brownies

Preparation time: 10 minutes | Cooking time: 30 minutes | Servings: 4

Ingredients:

¾ cup almond flour

½ tsp baking powder

½ tsp salt

¾ cup of coconut oil, melted

1 cups raw honey

2 tsp ground vanilla bean

3 eggs

1 tsp of cocoa powder

1 cup pumpkin puree

½ cup chopped pecans

¾ tsp ground cinnamon

½ tsp ground cloves

½ tsp ground nutmeg

Sprinkle with crushed pumpkin and sunflower seeds and hemp hearts

Directions:

Preheat oven to 350F and grease a baking pan.

Mix the almond flour, baking powder, and salt together in a bowl.

In another bowl, mix together the melted coconut oil, honey, and vanilla bean.

Beat in the eggs one at a time.

Slowly add the flour mixture and stir.

Add cocoa powder, pumpkin puree, pecans, cinnamon, cloves, and nutmeg.

Spread the batter into the bottom of the baking pan.

Bake until a toothpick inserted comes out clean, 45-50 minutes.

Cool in the pan, cut and serve.

Vegan sesame seeds cookies

Preparation time: 10 minutes | Cooking time: 25 minutes | Servings: 4

Ingredients:

1 cup toasted sesame seeds

2/3 cup almond flour

¼ cup raw honey

1/8 tsp baking powder

¼ cup of coconut oil (or tahini)

¼ cup of water

1 tbsp lemon juice

¼ tsp ground vanilla bean

Directions:

Heat oven to 350F.

Blend all ingredients until you get a sticky ball.

Make cookies and put them on the baking tray.

Bake for 20 minutes at 330F, until the cookies turn slightly brown.

Take them out and cool.

Coconut cream tart

Preparation time: 10 minutes | Cooking time: 30 minutes | Servings: 4

Ingredients:

Crust:

2 cups almonds, soaked overnight and drained

1 cup pitted dates, soaked overnight and drained

1 cup chopped dried apricots

1½ tsp ground vanilla bean

1 banana

Filling:

1 cup of flaked coconut

1 can of unsweetened coconut milk

¾ cup of raw honey

3 egg yolks

2 tbsp of arrowroot powder

2 tbsp of coconut oil

2 tsp of ground vanilla bean

1/8 tsp of salt

½ cup of coconut cream

Directions:

Heat the coconut milk, honey, salt and ground vanilla bean over medium heat in a medium-size saucepan.

In a separate bowl, whisk the egg yolks and arrowroot powder.

Add ½ cup of the warm coconut milk mixture to the egg yolks while whisking constantly.

Then pour the egg mixture back into the coconut milk mixture and whisk until the mix thickens and then mix for 3 more minutes.

Take off of the heat and mix in the coconut oil and flaked coconut.

Cool and pour in the tart crust and refrigerate.

Decorate with large coconut flakes.

Oatmeal raisin cookies

Preparation time: 10 minutes | Cooking time: 25 minutes | Servings: 4

Ingredients:

1 cup of coconut oil

1 cup of coconut sugar or raw honey

1½ cups almond flour

1 tsp salt

½ tsp grated nutmeg

1 tsp cinnamon

1½ cups raisins

2 large eggs, well beaten

1 tbsp ground vanilla bean

3 cups rolled oats

½ cup chopped walnuts

Directions:

Heat oven to 350F.

Grease cookie sheets with coconut oil or line with waxed or parchment paper.

Mix coconut oil, coconut sugar or raw honey in a large bowl and beat until fluffy.

Add vanilla.

Beat in eggs.

Mix almond flour, salt, cinnamon, and nutmeg in a separate bowl.

Stir these dry ingredients into a fluffy mixture.

Mix in raisins and nuts.

Mix in oats.

Spoon out on cookie sheets, leaving 2-inches between cookies.

Bake until edges turn golden brown.

Vegan superfoods granola

Preparation time: 10 minutes | Cooking time: 15 minutes | Servings: 4

Ingredients:

10 cup rolled oats

½ pound shredded coconut

2 cup raw sunflower seeds

1 cup sesame seeds or chia seeds

3 cup chopped nuts

1½ cup of water

1½ cup of coconut oil

1 cup raw honey

1½ tsp salt

2 tsp cinnamon

1 tbsp of ground vanilla bean

Dried cranberries

Directions:

Turn the oven on and heat oven to 300F.

Combine water, oil, raw honey, salt, cinnamon and vanilla in a large pan.

Heat until raw honey is dissolved, but don't boil.

Pour the honey over the dry ingredients and stir well.

Spread onto cookie sheets.

Bake 25-30 minutes, and stir occasionally.

Let it cool.

Store in a cool, dry place.

Vegan chocolate beet brownie

Preparation time: 10 minutes | Cooking time: 35 minutes | Servings: 4

Ingredients:

2 tbsp chia seeds

1¾ cups almond flour

¼ tsp baking soda

7 tbsp cocoa powder

4 ounces dark chocolate, chopped

1 tsp coffee

¾ tsp salt

¼ cup boiling water

1½ cups raw honey

6 tbsp coconut oil

1½ tsp ground vanilla bean

½ cup pecans, chopped

½ cup beet pulp – left over after juicing

Directions:

Preheat your oven to 350F.

Line a baking dish with parchment paper.

Mix together the almond flour and baking soda.

In another bowl mix the cocoa powder, chia seeds, chocolate, coffee and salt.

Add the boiling water and mix.

Add the honey, coconut oil, vanilla and flax meal mixture and blend.

Stir in the pecans and beet pulp.

Put the mix to a baking dish and bake.

Let cool and serve.

Vegan cacao chia cookies

Preparation time: 10 minutes | Cooking time: 35 minutes | Servings: 4

Ingredients:

4 tbsp of raw cacao powder

3 tbsp of chia seeds

1 cup of almonds

1 cup of cashews

1 cup of buckwheat flour

2 tbsp of coconut oil

1/3 of a cup of raw honey

¼ of a cup of dates

¼ of a cup of water

Directions:

Heat oven to 350F.

Blend all ingredients until you get a sticky ball.

Make cookies and put them on the baking tray.

Bake for 20 minutes at 350F, until the cookies turn slightly brown.

Take them out and cool.

Sweet superfoods pie crust

Preparation time: 10 minutes | Cooking time: 30 minutes | Servings: 4

Ingredients:

1 1/3 cups blanched almond flour

1/3 cup tapioca flour

½ tsp sea salt

1 large egg

¼ cup of coconut oil

2 tbsp coconut sugar or raw honey

1 tsp of ground vanilla bean

Directions:

Place almond flour, tapioca flour, sea salt, vanilla, egg and coconut sugar (if you use coconut sugar) in the bowl of a food processor.

Process 2-3 times to combine.

Add oil and sugar (or raw honey) and pulse with several one-second pulses and then let the food processor run until the mixture comes together.

Pour dough onto a sheet of plastic wrap.

Wrap and then press the dough into a 9-inch disk.

Refrigerate for 30 minutes.

Apple pie

Preparation time: 10 minutes | Cooking time: 35 minutes | Servings: 4

Ingredients:

For the crust:

See the previous recipe

For the apple filling:

2 tbsp coconut oil

9 sour apples, peeled, cored and cut into ¼-inch thick slices

¼ cup of coconut sugar or raw honey

½ tsp cinnamon

1/8 tsp sea salt

½ cup of coconut milk

For the topping:

1 cup ground nuts and seeds

Directions:

Filling: melt coconut oil in a large pot over medium heat.

Add apples, coconut sugar or raw honey, cinnamon and sea salt.

Increase heat to medium-high and cook, occasionally stirring, until apples release their moisture and sugar is melted.

Pour coconut milk or cream over apples and continue to cook until apples are soft and liquid has thickened, about 5 minutes, stirring occasionally.

Pour the filling into the crust and then top with topping.

Place a pie shield over the edges of the crust to avoid burning.

Bake until topping is just turning golden brown.

Cool and serve.

Vegan banana carrot bread

Preparation time: 10 minutes | Cooking time: 25 minutes | Servings: 4

Ingredients:

2 cups almond flour

1/3 cup raw honey

2 tsp cinnamon

2 tsp baking powder

½ tsp baking soda

Pinch of sea salt

2 tbsp hemp hearts

½ cup almond milk at the room temperature

¼ cup warmed coconut oil

3 mashed bananas

3 carrots, grated

¾ cup chopped walnuts

Directions:

Preheat oven to 350F.

In a large mixing bowl, add flour, honey, cinnamon, baking powder, soda and salt and mix well.

Add almond milk, coconut oil, hemp hearts, mashed bananas and mix.

Add carrots.

Greased loaf pan with coconut oil, pour the mixture and bake for 55-60 minutes.

Let cool for 10 minutes, remove from pan and let cool completely.

Store covered.

Serve warmed or at room temperature.

Slices would pair nicely with this sweet cashew cream.

Pumpkin pie

Preparation time: 10 minutes | Cooking time: 35 minutes | Servings: 4

Ingredients:

1½ cup homemade pumpkin puree

3 eggs

½ cup of coconut milk

½ cup raw honey

1 tbsp ground cinnamon

1 tsp Nutmeg

⅛ tsp sea salt

1 superfood sweet pie crust, 15 minutes prebaked

Directions:

In a food processor combine pumpkin puree and eggs.

Pulse in cinnamon, nutmeg, coconut milk, raw honey, and salt.

Pour filling into superfoods sweet pie crust and bake at 350F for 45 minutes.

Allow it to cool then refrigerate for 2 hours to set up.

Blueberry cream pie

Preparation time: 10 minutes | Cooking time: 30 minutes | Servings: 4

Ingredients:
Sweet superfoods pie crust filling:

2 tsp plant-based gelatin, dissolved in 2 tbsp hot water

1/3 cup lemon juice

1/3 cup raw honey

1 can coconut milk, chilled

4 cups blueberries for serving

Directions:

Mix the gelatin and water together.

Stir to dissolve and add the lemon juice.

Whip coconut milk and raw honey with electric mixer about 15 minutes.

Add the gelatin to the whipped cream.

Pour the filling into the crust.

Filling will set up in the refrigerator.

Chill for at 4 hours until set, and serve with lots of berries.

Rhubarb pie

Preparation time: 10 minutes | Cooking time: 35 minutes | Servings: 4

Ingredients:
Filling:

3 cups chopped rhubarb

¼ cup of water

1 cup raw honey

½ tsp sea salt

4 tbsp arrowroot powder

1/3 cup apple smoothie

2 tbsp coconut oil

¼ cup almond flour

1 tbsp lemon juice and 1 tsp grated zest

Crust:

See recipe for *Superfoods Pie Crust*

Directions:

Mix 2 cups of rhubarb, coconut oil, water, salt and ¾ cup honey and simmer over medium heat.

Preheat oven at 400F.

Mix ¼ cup honey, apple smoothie, ¼ cup almond flour and arrowroot powder.

Add this to the fruit mixture and stir well.

Continue to simmer for 2 more minutes.

Add 1 cup rhubarb and let the mixture cool.

Pour the mixture in the crust and bake at 375F for 40 minutes.

Chocolate cupcakes with matcha icing

Preparation time: 5 minutes | Cooking time: 40 minutes | Servings: 3

Ingredients:

150G self-raising flour

200g caster sugar

60g cocoa

½ tsp salt

½ tsp fine coffee espresso, decaf if liked

120ml milk

½ tsp vanilla concentrate

50ml vegetable oil

1 egg

120ml bubbling water

For the icing:

50g spread, at room temperature

50g icing sugar

1 tbsp matcha green tea powder

½ tsp vanilla bean glue

50g delicate cream cheddar

Directions:

Preheat the stove to 180C/160C fan.

Line a cupcake tin with paper or silicone cake cases.

Place the flour, sugar, cocoa, salt and coffee powder in a huge bowl and blend completely.

Add the milk, vanilla concentrate, vegetable oil and egg to the dry fixings and utilize an electric blender to beat until all-around joined.

Cautiously pour in the bubbling water gradually and beat on low speed until completely joined.

Utilize a rapid to beat for a further moment to add air to the hitter.

The player is significantly more fluid than an ordinary cake blend.

Spoon the player equally between the cake cases.

Each cake case ought to be close to ¾ full. Prepare in the broiler for 15-18 minutes, until the blend bobs back when tapped.

Expel from the broiler and permit to cool totally before icing.

To make the icing, cream the spread and icing sugar together until it's pale and smooth.

Include the matcha powder and vanillaand mix once more.

At long last include the cream cheddar and beat until smooth.

Funnel or spread over the cakes.

Upside down apple cake

Preparation time: 10 minutes | Cooking time: 35 minutes | Servings: 4

Ingredients:

Bottom fruit layer:

2 tbsp coconut oil, melted

1 apple, sliced, or ¼ cup blueberries, plums, banana etc.

2 tbsp walnut chunks 2 tbsp coconutsugar

1 tsp ground cinnamon.

2 eggs, beaten.

1/3 cup raw honey

¼ cup unsweetened coconut milk, or unsweetened almond milk.

1 tsp ground vanilla bean

1 tsp lemon juice.

1 banana, mashed, or ¼ cup blueberries

1/3 cup of coconut flour

Directions:

Heat the oven (350F), and grease a 9-inch cake pan.

Place 2 tbsp coconut oil into the cake pan, and put the pan into the preheated oven for a couple of minutes to melt oil. Make sure oil is evenly distributed all over the bottom of the pan.

Sprinkle 2 tbsp coconut sugar all over the oil.

Sprinkle 1 tsp cinnamon on top of the sweetened layer.

Layer apple slices or blueberries on top of the sweetened layer.

Add walnut pieces to fruit layer.

Set aside.

Combine all the "top cake layer" ingredients in a large mixing bowl except for the coconut flour.

Mix and add the coconut flour and mix well.

Spoon batter on top of fruit layer and spread evenly.

Bake until centre is set.

Remove from oven and let cool.

Slide a butter knife between cake and edge of pan to loosen cake.

Turn cake pan upside down onto a large plate or serving platter.

The cake should fall onto plate, but if not, then use a turning spatula to lift gently under cake a little, and then turn upside down onto the plate.

Black currants pie

Preparation time: 10 minutes | Cooking time: 30 minutes | Servings: 4

Ingredients:

Filling:

3 cups black currants

¼ cup of water

1 cup raw honey

½ tsp sea salt

4 tbsp arrowroot powder

1/3 cup apple smoothie

2 tbsp coconut oil

¼ cup almond flour

1 tbsp lemon juice and 1 tsp grated zest

Crust:

See recipe for *Superfoods Pie Crust*

Directions:

Mix 2 cups of black currants, coconut oil, water, salt and ¾ cup honey and simmer over medium heat.

Preheat oven at 400F.

Mix ¼ cup honey, apple smoothie, ¼ cup almond flour and arrowroot powder.

Add this to the fruit mixture and stir well.

Continue to simmer for 2 more minutes.

Add 1 cup black currants and let the mixture cool.

Pour the mixture in the crust and bake at 375F for 40 minutes.

Oats & blueberry cake

Preparation time: 10 minutes | Cooking time: 30 minutes | Servings: 4

Ingredients:

2½ cups old-fashioned rolled oats

1½ cups almond milk

1 beaten egg

1/3 cup raw honey

2 tbsp coconut oil

1 tsp ground vanilla bean

1 tsp ground cinnamon

1 tsp baking powder

¼ tsp salt

¾ cup blueberries

Directions:

Preheat oven to 375F.

Stir egg, honey, oil, vanilla, cinnamon, salt and baking powder into the oats until well combined.

Mix in blueberries.

Pour into the oiled pan.

Bake the oatmeal cake 25-30 minutes.

Let cool for 10 minutes.

Loosen and remove from the pan.

Top with blueberries and raspberries and serve warm.

Raspberry pie

Preparation time: 10 minutes | Cooking time: 25 minutes | Servings: 4

Ingredients:

Filling:

3 cups raspberries

¼ cup of water

1 cup raw honey

½ tsp sea salt

4 tbsp arrowroot powder

1/3 cup apple smoothie

2 tbsp coconut oil

¼ cup almond flour

1 tbsp lemon juice and 1 tsp grated zest

Crust:

See recipe for *Superfoods Pie Crust*

Directions:

Mix 2 cups of raspberry, coconut oil, water, salt and ¾ cup honey and simmer over medium heat.

Preheat oven at 400F.

Mix ¼ cup honey, apple smoothie, ¼ cup almond flour and arrowroot powder.

Add this to the fruit mixture and stir well.

Continue to simmer for 2 more minutes.

Add 1 cup raspberry and let the mixture cool.

Pour the mixture in the crust and bake at 375F for 40 minutes.

Honey chilli nuts

Preparation time: 10 minutes | Cooking time: 15 minutes | Servings: 4

Ingredients:

150G (5oz) walnuts

150G (5oz) pecan nuts

50g (2oz) softened butter

1 tbsp honey

½ bird's eye chilli, very finely chopped and de-seeded

Directions:

Preheat the oven to 180C/360F.

Combine the butter, honey and chilli in a bowl then add the nuts and stir them well.

Spread the nuts onto a lined baking sheet and roast them in the oven for 10 minutes, stirring once halfway through.

Remove from the oven and allow them to cool before eating.

Homemade hummus & celery

Preparation time: 10 minutes | Cooking time: 25 minutes | Servings: 4

Ingredients:

8 sticks of celery, cut into batons

175G (6oz) tinned chickpeas (garbanzo beans), drained

2 cloves of garlic, crushed

1 tbsp fresh parsley, chopped

1 tbsp tahini (sesame seed paste) juice of lemon

1 tbsp olive oil

Directions:

Place the chickpeas (garbanzo beans) into a blender along with the garlic, tahini paste and lemon juice.

Process until it's smooth and creamy.

Transfer the mixture to a serving bowl.

Make a small well in the centre of the dip and pour in the olive oil.

Sprinkle with parsley.

Serve the celery sticks on a plate alongside the hummus.

Watermelon juice

Preparation time: 10 minutes | Cooking time: 0 minutes | Servings: 4

Ingredients:
20g of young kale leaves

250G of watermelon chunks

4 mint leaves

½ cucumber

Directions:
Remove the stalks from the kale and roughly chop it.

Peel the cucumber, if preferred, and then halve it and seed it.

Place all ingredients in a blender or juicer and process until you achieve the desired consistency.

Serve immediately.

Berries banana smoothie

Preparation time: 10 minutes | Cooking time: 35 minutes | Servings: 2

Ingredients:
½ cup of coconut milk

1½ cups of mixed berries (strawberries and blueberries) - could be frozen or fresh

¾ cup of water

4 ice cubes

1 tbsp of molasses

1 banana

Directions:
Place all the ingredients in a blender and blend until smooth.

You can add water to the smoothie until you achieve your desired consistency, then serve.

Pomegranate guacamole

Preparation time: 10 minutes | Cooking time: 35 minutes

Ingredients:
The flesh of 2 ripe avocados

seeds from 1 pomegranate

1 bird's eye chilli pepper, finely chopped

½ red onion, finely chopped

juice of 1 lime

Directions:
Place the avocado, onion, chilli and lime juice into a blender and process until smooth.

Stir in the pomegranate seeds.

Chill before serving.

Serve as a dip for chop vegetables.

Tofu guacamole

Preparation time: 10 minutes | Cooking time: 35 minutes

Ingredients:

225g (8oz) silken tofu

3 avocados

2 tbsp fresh coriander (cilantro) chopped

1 bird's eye chilli

Juice of 1 lime

Directions:

Place all of the ingredients into a food processor and blend a soft chunky consistency.

Serve with crudités.

Ginger & turmeric tea

Preparation time: 10 minutes | Cooking time: 35 minutes

Ingredients:

2.5cm (1-inch) chunk fresh ginger root, peeled

¼ tsp turmeric

1 tsp of honey (optional) hot water

Directions:

Make incisions in the piece of root ginger, without cutting all the way through.

Place the ginger and turmeric in a cup and pour in hot water.

Allow it to steep for 7 minutes.

Add a tsp of honey if you wish.

Sirtfood green juice

Preparation time: 10 minutes | Cooking time: 35 minutes | Servings: 1

Ingredients:

2 large handfuls kale

5g of parsley

½ green apple

2-3 large stalks green celery plus the leaves

A large handful rocket (about 30g)

Juice of ½ lemon

½ level tsp matcha green tea

A very small handful of lovage leaves (optional)

Directions:

Simply mix all the greens – rocket, parsley, kale and lovage using a juicer, just fully juice them.

Your target is to juice around 50ml from the greens.

Next step is to add the green apple and the celery.

Simply squeeze the lemon into the juice.

Most likely, you will have more than 250ML of juice at this stage.

When ready to consume, pour into a glass and you can now add your matcha green tea powder.

Stir and enjoy!

Suggestion: for night drinking, you can forego the matcha green tea, note that tea contains caffeine, and you might find it harder to sleep at night after your green juice.

Special green tea smoothie

Preparation time: 10 minutes | Cooking time: 35 minutes | Servings: 2

Ingredients:

250 ml of milk

2 ripe bananas

½ tsp vanilla bean paste

2 tsp of honey

6 ice cubes

2 tsp of matcha green tea powder

Directions:

Mix all the ingredients together using a blender or smoothie machine.

Serve and enjoy.

Special blackcurrant and oat yoghurt

Preparation time: 10 minutes | Cooking time: 30 minutes | Servings: 4

Ingredients:

400g of Greek yoghurt, plain

200g blackcurrants washed and stalks removed

200 ml of water

4 tbsp of caster sugar (or your own choice of sweetener)

80g of oats

Directions:

In a small pan, simply place the blackcurrants, water and sugar.

Bring to boil.

After boiling, slightly reduce the heat, maintain the simmer and cook for another 4-5 minutes.

Turn the heat off and let the mixture cool.

After cooling, you can now refrigerate your blackcurrant compote until ready to be used.

Using a large bowl, place the yoghurt and oats, then thoroughly stir in together.

Divide the blackcurrant compote into 4 serving bowls, then just simple top with the oats and yoghurt.

Mix and enjoy.

The Asian style king prawn stir fry with buckwheat noodles

Preparation time: 10 minutes | Cooking time: 25 minutes | Servings: 3-4

Ingredients:

300g shelled raw king prawns, deveined

4 tsp soy sauce or tamari

4 tsp of extra virgin olive oil

150G of buckwheat noodles

2 garlic clove, finely chopped

2 bird's eye chillies, finely chopped

2 tsp finely chopped fresh ginger

40g red onions, sliced

80g celery, trimmed and sliced

150G green beans, chopped

100g kale, roughly chopped

200ml chicken stock

10g of celery leaves

Directions:

Over high heat place the frying pan and cook the prawns in 2 tsp of tamari and 2 tsp of extra virgin olive oil for about 3 minutes.

Once cooked, carefully transfer the prawns to a plate and set aside.

Simply follow the direction on the packet and cook the noodles in boiling water.

Estimated time is about 5 minutes or as directed.

Carefully drain and set the noodles aside.

Over medium-high heat, sauté the garlic, red onion, ginger, chillies, celery, kale and beans using the remaining oil.

Do this for about 2 minutes, then add the stock and bring to boil.

After boiling, let it simmer for another 2 minutes or until the veggies are cooked (the crunchiness should still be preserved).

Add the noodles, prawns, celery leaves to the pan and bring to a boil.

Serve and enjoy.

Simple tofu scrambled for breakfast

Preparation time: 10 minutes | Cooking time: 30 minutes | Servings: 4

Ingredients:

Tofu scrambled:

16 ounces of extra firm tofu

4 cups kale, loosely chopped

½ red onion, thinly sliced

1 red pepper, thinly sliced

Extra virgin olive oil

Sauce:

1 tsp garlic powder

1 tsp cumin powder

½ tsp chilli powder

1 tsp sea salt

½ tsp turmeric (optional)

Directions:

Make sure that the tofu is drained.

You can do this using an absorbent towel with a skillet on top.

Do this for about 10-15 minutes.

In a small bowl, prepare the sauce by adding all the dry spices then add enough water for it to become a pourable sauce.

Set aside.

Over medium heat, use a large skillet, and add about 2 tbsp of extra virgin olive oil once the skillet is hot.

Add the red pepper and onion then season with salt and pepper.

Stir and cook for about 3-5 minutes.

Add the kale and season to taste with salt and pepper.

Cover it for another 2 mins.

Unwrap the tofu then crumble into bite-sizes using a fork or a spoon.

Move the veggies on one side of the pan, then add the tofu to the clear spot.

Sauté for about 2-3 minutes then pour in the sauce over the tofu.

Stir and cook until the tofu is lightly browned.

Serve and enjoy.

You can also add more sirtuin-rich food on the side.

Iced cranberry green tea

Preparation time: 10 minutes | Cooking time: 35 minutes

Ingredients:

150Ml (5 fl oz) light cranberry juice

100ml (3½ fl oz) green tea, cooled

A squeeze of lemon juice a handful of crushed ice (optional) sprig of mint

Directions:

Pour the green tea and cranberry into a glass and add a squeeze of lemon juice.

Top it off with some ice and garnish with a mint leaf.

Chapter 10: Main Dishes

Coq au vin

Preparation time: 10 minutes | Cooking time: 40 minutes | Serving: 2

Ingredients:

450g (1Lb) button mushrooms

100g (3½oz) streaky bacon, chopped

16 chicken thighs, skin removed

3 cloves of garlic, crushed

3 tbsp fresh parsley, chopped

3 carrots, chopped

2 red onions, chopped 2 tbsp plain flour

2 tbsp olive oil

750ml (1¼ pints) red wine 1 bouquet garni

Directions:

Place the flour on a large plate and coat the chicken in it.

Heat the olive oil in a large saucepan, add the chicken and brown it, before setting aside.

Fry the bacon in the pan then add the onion and cook for 5 minutes.

Pour in the red wine and add the chicken, carrots, bouquet garni and garlic.

Transfer it to a large ovenproof dish.

Cook in the oven at 180C/360F for 1 hour.

Remove the bouquet garni and skim off any excess fat, if necessary.

Add in the mushrooms and cook for 15 minutes.

Stir in the parsley just before serving.

Kale white bean pork soup

Preparation time: 5 minutes | Cooking time: 45 minutes | Servings: 4-6

Ingredients:

3 tbsp extra-virgin olive oil

3 tbsp chilli powder

1 tbsp jalapeno hot sauce

2 pounds bone-in pork chops

Salt

4 stalks celery, chopped

1 large white onion, chopped

3 cloves garlic, chopped

2 cups chicken broth

2 cups diced tomatoes

2 cups cooked white beans

6 cups packed kale

Directions:

Preheat the broiler.

Whisk hot sauce, 1 tbsp olive oil and chilli powder in a bowl.

Season the pork chops with ½ tsp salt.

Rub chops with the spice mixture on both sides and place them on a rack set over a baking sheet.

Set aside.

Heat 1 tbsp olive oil in a pot over medium heat.

Add the celery, garlic, onion and the remaining 2 tbsp chilli powder.

Cook until onions are translucent, stirring (approx. 8 minutes).

Add tomatoes and the chicken broth to the pot. Cook and occasionally stir until reduced by about one-third (approx. 7 minutes).

Add the kale and the beans.

Reduce the heat to medium, cover and cook until the kale is tender (approx. 7minutes).

Add up to ½ cup of water if the mixture looks dry and season with salt.

In the meantime, broil the pork until browned (approx. 4 to 6 minutes).

Flip and broil until cooked through.

Serve with the kale and beans.

Turkey satay skewers

Preparation time: 5 minutes | Cooking time: 30 minutes | Servings: 3

Ingredients:

250G (9oz) turkey breast, cubed

25G (1oz) smooth peanut butter

1 clove of garlic, crushed

½ small bird's eye chilli (or more if you like it hotter), finely chopped

½ tsp ground turmeric

200ml (7fl oz) coconut milk

2 tsp soy sauce

Directions: Combine the coconut milk, peanut butter, turmeric, soy sauce, garlic and chilli. Add the turkey pieces to the bowl and stir them until they are completely coated. Push the turkey onto metal skewers.

Place the satay skewers on a barbeque or under a hot grill (broiler) and cook for 4-5 minutes on each side, until they are completely cooked.

Salmon & capers

Preparation time: 5 minutes | Cooking time: 40 minutes | Servings: 3

Ingredients:

75g (3oz) Greek yoghurt

4 salmon fillets, skin removed

4 tsp dijon mustard

1 tbsp capers, chopped

2 tsp fresh parsley

Zest of 1 lemon

Directions:

In a bowl, mix together the yoghurt, mustard, lemon zest, parsley and capers.

Thoroughly coat the salmon in the mixture.

Place the salmon under a hot grill (broiler) and cook for 3-4 minutes on each side, or until the fish is cooked.

Serve with mashed potatoes and vegetables or a large green leafy salad.

Moroccan chicken casserole

Preparation time: 5 minutes | Cooking time: 20 minutes | Servings: 3

Ingredients:

250G (9oz) tinned chickpeas (garbanzo beans) drained

4 chicken breasts, cubed

4 Medjool dates halved

6 dried apricots, halved

1 red onion, sliced

1 carrot, chopped

1 tsp ground cumin

1 tsp ground cinnamon

1 tsp ground turmeric

1 bird's eye chilli, chopped

600ml (1 pint) chicken stock (broth)

25g (1oz) cornflour

60ml (2fl oz) water

2 tbsp fresh coriander

Directions:

Place the chicken, chickpeas (garbanzo beans), onion, carrot, chilli, cumin, turmeric, cinnamon and stock (broth) into a large saucepan.

Bring it to the boil, reduce the heat and simmer for 25 minutes.

Add in the dates and apricots and simmer for 10 minutes.

In a cup, mix the cornflour together with the water until it becomes a smooth paste.

Pour the mixture into the saucepan and stir until it thickens.

Add in the coriander (cilantro) and mix well.

Serve with buckwheat or couscous.

Vegetable broth

Preparation time: 5 minutes | Cooking time: 40 minutes | Servings: 6 cups

Ingredients:

1 tbsp olive oil

1 large red onion

2 stalks celery, including some leaves

2 large carrots

1 bunch green onions, chopped

8 cloves garlic, minced

8 sprigs fresh parsley

6 sprigs fresh thyme

2 bay leaves

1 tsp salt

2 quarts water

Directions:

Chop veggies into small chunks.

Heat oil in a soup pot, add onion, scallions, celery, carrots, garlic, parsley, thyme, and bay leaves.

Cook over high heat for 5 to 7 minutes, stirring occasionally.

Bring to a boil and add salt.

Lower heat and simmer, uncovered, for 30 minutes.

Strain.

Other ingredients to consider: broccoli stalk, celery root

Chicken broth

Preparation time: 5 minutes | Cooking time: 50 minutes | Servings: 3

Ingredients:

4lbs. fresh chicken (wings, necks, backs, legs, bones)

2 peeled onions or 1 cup chopped leeks

2 celery stalks

1 carrot

8 black peppercorns

2 sprigs fresh thyme

2 sprigs fresh parsley

1 tsp salt

Directions:

Put cold water in a stockpot and add chicken.

Bring just to a boil.

Skim any foam from the surface.

Add other ingredients, return just to a boil, and reduce heat to a slow simmer.

Simmer for 2 hours.

Let cool to warm room temperature and strain.

Keep chilled and use or freeze broth within a few days.

Before using, defrost and boil.

Beef broth

Preparation time: 5 minutes | Cooking time: 40 minutes | Servings: 3

Ingredients:

4-5 pounds beef bones and few veal bones

1 pound of stew meat (chuck or flank steak) cut into 2-inch chunks

Olive oil

1-2 medium red onions, peeled and quartered

1-2 large carrots, cut into 1-2-inch segments

1 celery rib, cut into 1-inch segments

2-3 cloves of garlic, unpeeled

A handful of parsley stems and leaves

1-2 bay leaves

10 peppercorns

Directions:

Heat oven to 375F.

Rub olive oil over the stew meat pieces, carrots, and onions.

Place stew meat or beef scraps, stock bones, carrots and onions in a large roastingpan.

Roast in the oven for about 45 minutes, turning everything halfway through the cooking.

Place everything from the oven in a large stockpot.

Pour some boiling water in the oven pan and scrape up all of the browned bits and pour all in the stockpot.

Add parsley, celery, garlic, bay leaves, and peppercorns to the pot.

Fill the pot with cold water, to 1-inch over the top of the bones.

Bring the stockpot to a regular simmer and then reduce the heat to low, so it just barely simmers. Cover the pot loosely and let simmer low and slow for 3-4 hours.

Scoop away the fat and any scum that rises to the surface once in a while.

After cooking, remove the bones and vegetables from the pot.

Strain the broth.

Let cool to room temperature and then put in the refrigerator.

The fat will solidify once the broth has chilled.

Discard the fat (or reuse it) and pour the broth into a jar and freeze it.

Chilli con Carne

Preparation time: 5 minutes | Cooking time: 30 minutes | Servings: 3

Ingredients:

450g (1Lb) lean minced beef

400g (14oz) chopped tomatoes

200g (7oz) red kidney beans

2 tbsp tomato purée

2 cloves of garlic, crushed

2 red onions, chopped

2 bird's eye chillies, finely chopped

1 red pepper (bell pepper), chopped

1 stick of celery, finely chopped

1 tbsp cumin

1 tbsp turmeric

1 tbsp cocoa powder

400ml (14 fl oz) beef stock (broth)

175ML (6fl oz) red wine

1 tbsp olive oil

Directions:

Heat the oil in a large saucepan, add the onion and cook for 5 minutes.

Add in the garlic, celery, chilli, turmeric, and cumin and cook for 2 minutes before adding then meat then cook for another 5 minutes.

Pour in the stock (broth), red wine, tomatoes, tomato purée, red pepper (bell pepper), kidney beans and cocoa powder.

Simmer on low heat for 45 minutes, keep it covered and stirring occasionally.

Serve with brown rice or buckwheat.

Prawn & coconut curry

Preparation time: 5 minutes | Cooking time: 35 minutes | Servings: 3

Ingredients:

400g (14oz) tinned chopped tomatoes

400g (14oz) large prawns (shrimps), shelled and raw

25G (1OZ) fresh coriander (cilantro) chopped

3 red onions, finely chopped

3 cloves of garlic, crushed

2 bird's eye chillies

½ tsp ground coriander (cilantro)

½ tsp turmeric

400ml (14fl oz) coconut milk

1 tbsp olive oil

Juice of 1 lime

Directions:

Place the onions, garlic, tomatoes, chillies, lime juice, turmeric, ground coriander (cilantro), chillies and half of the fresh coriander (cilantro) into a blender and blitz until you have a smooth curry paste.

Heat the olive oil in a frying pan, add the paste and cook for 2 minutes.

Stir in the coconut milk and warm it thoroughly.

Add the prawns (shrimps) to the paste and cook them until they have turned pink and are completely cooked.

Stir in the fresh coriander (cilantro).

Serve with rice.

Chicken & bean casserole

Preparation time: 5 minutes | Cooking time: 40 minutes | Servings: 3

Ingredients:

400g (14oz) chopped tomatoes

400g (14oz) tinned cannellini beans or haricot beans

8 chicken thighs, skin removed

2 carrots, peeled and finely chopped

2 red onions, chopped

4 sticks of celery

4 large mushrooms

2 red peppers (bell peppers), de-seeded and chopped

1 clove of garlic

2 tbsp soy sauce

1 tbsp olive oil

1.75 litres (3 pints) chicken stock (broth)

Directions:

Heat the olive oil in a saucepan, add the garlic and onions and cook for 5 minutes.

Add in the chicken and cook for 5 minutes then add the carrots, cannellini beans, celery, red peppers (bell peppers) and mushrooms.

Pour in the stock (broth) soy sauce and tomatoes.

Bring it to the boil, reduce the heat and simmer for 45 minutes.

Serve with rice or new potatoes.

Sesame miso chicken

Preparation time: 5 minutes | Cooking time: 40 minutes | Servings: 3

Ingredients: 1 skinless cod fillet

½ cup buckwheat ½ red onion, sliced

2 stalks celery, sliced 10 green beans

2 cups kale, roughly chopped

3 sprigs of parsley

1 garlic clove, finely chopped

1 pinch cayenne or ½ chilli

1 tsp finely chopped fresh ginger

1 tsp Sesame seeds 2 tsp of miso

1 tbsp mirin/rice wine vinegar

1 tbsp extra virgin olive oil

1 tbsp of soy sauce 1 tsp ground turmeric

Directions:

Coat the cod with a mixture of the miso, mirin and 1 tsp of the oil and set aside for 30 minutes up to one hour in the refrigerator.

Heat the oven to 400F, then bake the cod for 10 minutes.

Sautee the onion and stir-fry in the oil that remains along with the green beans, kale, celery, chilli pepper, garlic, ginger.

Sautee until the kale is wilted, but the beans and celery are tender.

Add dashes of water if needed to the pan as you go.

Cook the buckwheat according to the packet directions with the turmeric for 3 minutes.

Add the sesame seeds, parsley and tamari to the stir-fry and serve with the greens and fish.

Tofu and curry

Preparation time: 5 minutes | Cooking time: 36 minutes | Servings: 4

Ingredients:

8 oz dried lentils (red preferably)

1 cup boiling water

1 cup frozen edamame (soy) beans

7 oz (½ of most packages) firm tofu, chopped into cubes

2 tomatoes, chopped 1 lime juices

5-6 kale leaves, stalks removed and torn

1 large onion, chopped

4 cloves garlic, peeled and grated

1 large chunk of ginger, grated

½ red chilli pepper, deseeded (use less if too much)

½ tsp ground turmeric

¼ tsp cayenne pepper 1 tsp paprika

½ tsp ground cumin 1 tsp salt

1 tbsp olive oil

Directions: Add the onion, sauté in the oil for few minutes then add the chilli, garlic and ginger for a bit longer until wilted but not burned. Add the seasonings, then the lentils and stir.

Add in the boiling water and cook for 10 minutes.

Simmer for up to 30 minutes longer, so it will be stew-like but not overly mushy.

You should check the texture of the lentils halfway though.

Add tomato, tofu and edamame, then lime juice and kale.

Test for when the kale is tender, and then it is ready to serve.

Chicken and kale with spicy salsa

Preparation time: 5 minutes | Cooking time: 40 minutes | Servings: 1

Ingredients:

1 skinless, boneless chicken filet/breast

¼ cup buckwheat

¼ lemon, juiced

1 tbsp Extra virgin olive oil

1 cup kale, chopped

½ red onion, sliced

1 tsp fresh ginger, chopped

2 tsp ground turmeric salsa:

1 tomato

3 sprigs of parsley, chopped

1 tbsp chopped capers

1 chilli, deseeded and minced (use less if desired)

juice of ¼ lemon

Directions:

Chop all ingredients above, just for the salsa, and set aside in a bowl.

Pre-eat the oven to 425F.

Add 1 tsp of the turmeric, the lemon juice and a little oil to the chicken, cover and set aside for 10 minutes.

In a hot pan, slide the chicken and marinade and cook for 2-3 minutes each side, on high to sear it.

Then, slide it all onto a baking-safe dish and cook for about 20 minutes or until cooked (testing for pinkness).

Lightly steam the kale in a steamer, or on the stovetop with a lid and some water, for about 5 minutes.

You want to wilt the kale, not boil or burn it.

Sautee the red onions and ginger, and after 4-5 minutes, add the cooked kale and stir for 1 minute.

Cook the buckwheat, adding in the turmeric (see the package or look online if it was bought in bulk, for cooking directions).

Serve the chicken along with the buckwheat, kale, and spicy salsa.

Smoked salmon sirt salad

Preparation time: 5 minutes | Cooking time: 45 minutes | Servings: 3

Ingredients:

1 cup, or ¼ package (if large) of smoked salmon slices (no cooking needed!)

1 avocado, pitted, sliced, and scooped out

10 walnuts, chopped

5 lovage (or celery leaves), chopped

2 celery stalks, chopped or sliced thinly

½ small red onion, sliced thinly

1 Medjool pitted date, chopped

1 tbsp capers

1 tbsp extra virgin olive oil

¼ of a lemon, juiced

5 sprigs of parsley, chopped

Directions:

Wash and dry salad makings and vegetables, top with salmon.

Lentil lovage salad

Preparation time: 5 minutes | Cooking time: 40 minutes | Servings: 1

Ingredients:

1 cup cooked red lentils (prepare in advance, use warmed or at room temperature)

1 avocado, pitted, sliced, and scoopedout

2 cups baby kale, chopped

2 celery stalks, chopped or sliced thinly

½ small red onion, sliced thinly

1 Medjool pitted date, chopped

¼ cup red currants

1 tsp turmeric

1 tbsp extra virgin olive oil

¼ of a lemon, juiced

5 sprigs of parsley, chopped

Directions:

Add ingredients and toss together gently. Serve.

Chicken, kale and lentil soup

Preparation time: 5 minutes | Cooking time: 25 minutes | Servings: 3

Ingredients:

5 cups of chicken or vegetablestocks

1 chicken breast, chopped (good use for any leftover chicken form other recipes!)

1 small red onion

2 cups of kale, finelychopped

1 cup of spinach, chopped

1 cup of lentils

1 celery stick, chopped

1 carrot, chopped

1 small chilli pepper or a dash of cayenne

A dash of salt

1 tsp of extra virgin olive oil

Directions:

Cook the lentils according to the package, but taking them out just a few minutes before they would be done.

Set aside.

Add the vegetables to a large pot, sauté in a bit of the oil on medium heat.

Stir until the vegetables are softer but not cooked through.

Add the chicken (precooked and leftover, plain, skinless chicken), add the lentil you had set aside, and cook for 3-5 minutes more.

Add a dash of the salt.

Add the stock, turn down to low, and simmer for 20 minutes.

Remove from heat.

Serve when cooled.

Spicy Asian noodle soup

Preparation time: 5 minutes | Cooking time: 40 minutes | Servings: 2

Ingredients:

1 package buckwheat noodles, prepared as instructed on package

1 small red onion

2 stalks of celery, washed and chopped

1 chunk of ginger, diced

1 clove of garlic, minced

1 cup of arugula

¼ cup basil leaves, wash, dry and then chop

¼ cup of walnuts

1 tsp of sesame seeds

2 tbsp Blackcurrants

½ chilli pepper

5 cups of chicken or vegetable stock

Juice of ½ lime

1 tsp extra virgin olive oil

1 tbsp of soy sauce

Directions:

Cook the noodles as instructed and set aside.

In a pan, sauté all of the vegetables, ginger, garlic, chilli, and nuts for about 10 minutes on very low heat.

Add the stock, and simmer for another 5 minutes.

Cut the noodles (roughly) so that they are a size, small enough to eat in a soup comfortably.

Add these to the stock, toss in the sesame seeds, lime juice and remove from heat.

Cool and serve.

Mussels in red wine sauce

Preparation time: 5 minutes | Cooking time: 20 minutes | Servings: 3

Ingredients:

800g (2Lb) mussels

2 x 400g (14oz) tins of chopped tomatoes

25G (1OZ) butter

1 tbsp fresh chives, chopped

1 tbsp fresh parsley, chopped

1 bird's eye chilli, finely chopped

4 cloves of garlic, crushed

400ml (14fl oz) red wine

Juice of 1 lemon

Directions:

Wash the mussels, remove their beards and set them aside.

Heat the butter in a large saucepan and add in the red wine.

Reduce the heat and add the parsley, chives, chilli and garlic whilst stirring.

Add in the tomatoes, lemon juice and mussels.

Cover the saucepan and cook for 2-3.remove the saucepan from the heat and take out any mussels which haven't opened and discard them.

Serve and eat immediately.

Roast balsamic vegetables

Preparation time: 5 minutes | Cooking time: 40 minutes | Servings: 3

Ingredients:

4 tomatoes, chopped

2 red onions, chopped

3 sweet potatoes, peeled and chopped

100g (3½ oz) red chicory (or if unavailable, use yellow)

100g (3½ oz) kale, finely chopped

300g (11oz) potatoes, peeled and chopped

5 stalks of celery, chopped

1 bird's eye chilli, de-seeded and finely chopped

2 tbsp fresh parsley, chopped

2 tbsp fresh coriander (cilantro) chopped

3 tbsp olive oil

2 tbsp balsamic vinegar

1 tsp mustard

Sea salt

Freshly ground black pepper

Directions:

Place the olive oil, balsamic, mustard, parsley and coriander (cilantro) into abowl and mix well.

Toss all the remaining ingredients into the dressing and season with salt and pepper.

Transfer the vegetables to an ovenproof dish and cook in the oven at 200C/400F for 45 minutes.

Tomato & goat's cheese pizza

Preparation time: 5 minutes | Cooking time: 40 minutes | Servings: 3

Ingredients:

225g (8oz) buckwheat flour

2 tsp dried yeast

Pinch of salt

150Ml (5fl oz) slightly water

1 tsp olive oil

For the topping:

75g (3oz) feta cheese, crumbled

75g (3oz) passata (or tomato paste)

1 tomato, sliced

1 red onion, finely chopped

25G (1oz) rocket (arugula) leaves, chopped

Directions:

In a bowl, combine all the ingredients for the pizza dough then allow it to stand for at least an hour until it has doubled in size.

Roll the dough out to a size to suit you.

Spoon the passata onto the base and add the rest of the toppings.

Bake in the oven at 200C/400F for 15-20 minutes or until browned at the edges and crispy and serve.

Tofu Thai curry

Preparation time: 5 minutes | Cooking time: 30 minutes | Servings: 3

Ingredients:

400g (14oz) tofu, diced

200g (7oz) sugar snap peas

5cm (2-inch) chunk fresh ginger root, peeled and finely chopped

2 red onions, chopped

2 cloves of garlic, crushed

2 bird's eye chillies

2 tbsp tomato puree

1 stalk of lemongrass, inner stalks only

1 tbsp fresh coriander (cilantro), chopped

1 tsp cumin

300ml (½ pint) coconut milk

200ml (7fl oz) vegetable stock (broth)

1 tbsp virgin olive oil

juice of 1 lime

Directions:

Heat the oil in a frying pan, add the onion and cook for 4 minutes.

Add in the chillies, cumin, ginger, and garlic and cook for 2 minutes.

Add the tomato puree, lemongrass, sugar-snap peas, lime juice and tofu and cook for 2 minutes.

Pour in the stock (broth), coconut milk and coriander (cilantro) and simmer for 5 minutes.

Serve with brown rice or buckwheat and a handful of rocket (arugula) leaves on the side.

Tender spiced lamb

Preparation time: 5 minutes | Cooking time: 40 minutes | Servings: 3

Ingredients:

1.35kg (3lb) lamb shoulder

3 red onions, sliced

3 cloves of garlic, crushed

1 bird's eye chilli, finely chopped

1 tsp turmeric

1 tsp ground cumin

½ tsp ground coriander (cilantro)

¼ tsp ground cinnamon

2 tbsp olive oil

Directions:

In a bowl, combine the chilli, garlic and spices with a tbsp of olive oil.

Coat the lamb with the spice mixture and marinate it for an hour, or overnight if you can.

Heat the remaining oil in a pan, add the lamb and brown it for 3-4 minutes on all sides to seal it.

Place the lamb in an ovenproof dish. Add in the red onions and cover the dish withfoil.

Transfer to the oven and roast at 170C/325F for 4 hours.

The lamb should be extremely tender and falling off the bone.

Serve with rice or couscous, salad or vegetables.

Chilli cod fillets

Preparation time: 5 minutes | Cooking time: 10 minutes | Servings: 3

Ingredients:

4 cod fillets (approx 150g each)

2 tbsp fresh parsley, chopped

2 bird's eye chillies (or more if you like it hot)

2 cloves of garlic, chopped

4 tbsp olive oil

Directions:

Heat a tbsp of olive oil in a frying pan, add the fish and cook for 7-8 minutes or until thoroughly cooked, turning once halfway through.

Remove and keep warm.

Pour the remaining olive oil into the pan and add the chilli, chopped garlic and parsley.

Warm it thoroughly.

Serve the fish onto plates and pour the warm chilli oil over it.

Steak & mushroom noodles

Preparation time: 5 minutes | Cooking time: 30 minutes | Servings: 3

Ingredients:

100g (3½oz) shitake mushrooms, halved, if large

100g (3½oz) chestnut mushrooms, sliced

150G (5oz) udon noodles

75g (3oz) kale, finely chopped

75g (3oz) baby leaf spinach, chopped

2 sirloin steaks

2 tbsp miso paste

2.5cm (1In) piece fresh ginger, finely chopped

2 tbsp olive oil

1 star anise

1 red chilli, finely sliced

1 red onion, finely chopped

1 tbsp fresh coriander (cilantro) chopped

1 litre (1½ pints) warm water

Directions:

Pour the water into a saucepan and add in the miso, star anise and ginger.

Bring it to the boil, reduce the heat and simmer gently.

In the meantime, cook the noodles according to their directions then drain them.

Heat the oil in a saucepan, add the steak and cook for around 2-3 minutes on each side (or 1-2 minutes, for rare meat) remove the meat and set aside.

Place the mushrooms, spinach, coriander (cilantro) and kale into the miso broth and cook for 5 minutes.

In the meantime, heat the remaining oil in a separate pan and fry the chilli and onion for 4 minutes, until softened.

Serve the noodles into bowls and pour the soup on top.

Thinly slice the steaks and add them to the top.

Serve immediately.

Roast lamb & red wine sauce

Preparation time: 5 minutes | Cooking time: 20 minutes | Servings: 3

Ingredients:

1.5Kg (3lb 6oz) leg of lamb

5 cloves of garlic

6 sprigs of rosemary

3 tbsp parsley

1 tbsp honey

1 tbsp olive oil

½ tsp sea salt

300ml (½ pint) red wine

Directions:

Place the rosemary, garlic, parsley and salt into a pestle and mortar or small bowl and blend the ingredients together.

Make small slits in the lamb and press a little of the mixture into each incision.

Pour the oil over the meat and cover it with foil.

Roast in the oven for around 1 hour 20 minutes.

Pour the wine into a small saucepan and stir in the honey.

Warm the liquid then reduce the heat and simmer until reduced.

Once the lamb is ready, pour the sauce over it, then return it to the oven to cook for another 5 minutes.

Cannellini & spinach curry

Preparation time: 5 minutes | Cooking time: 40 minutes | Servings: 3

Ingredients:

400g (14oz) cannellini beans

400g (14oz) tinned tomatoes

150G (5oz) cauliflower florets

75g (3oz) spinach

1 red onion, chopped

1 carrot, chopped

3 cloves of garlic, chopped

1 tsp ground cumin

1½ tsp turmeric

1 tsp curry powder

1 bird's eye chilli, finely chopped

600ml (1 pint) vegetable stock (broth)

2 tbsp olive oil

Directions:

Heat the oil in a saucepan.

Add the onion, cauliflower, carrots and garlic and cook for 5 minutes until the vegetables soften.

Add the cumin, turmeric, curry powder and chilli and stir for 2 minutes.

Add the tomatoes, cannellini beans and stock (broth).

Bring to the boil, reduce the heat and simmer for 25-30 minutes.

Stir in the spinach for the last two minutes of cooking, until it has wilted.

Serve with brown rice.

Turkey curry

Preparation time: 5 minutes | Cooking time: 40 minutes | Servings: 3

Ingredients:

450g (1Lb), turkey breasts, chopped

100g (3½ oz) fresh rocket (arugula) leaves

5 cloves garlic, chopped

3 tsp medium curry powder

2 tsp turmeric powder

2 tbsp fresh coriander (cilantro), finely chopped

2 bird's eye chillies, chopped

2 red onions, chopped

400ml (14fl oz) full-fat coconut milk

2 tbsp olive oil

Directions:

Heat the olive oil in a saucepan, add the chopped red onions and cook them for around 5 minutes or until soft.

Stir in the garlic and the turkey and cook it for 7-8 minutes.

Stir in the turmeric, chillies and curry powder then add the coconut milk and coriander (cilantro).

Bring it to the boil, reduce the heat and simmer for around 10 minutes.

Scatter the rocket (arugula) onto plates and spoon the curry on top.

Serve alongside brown rice.

King prawn stir-fry & soba

Preparation time: 5 minutes | Cooking time: 50 minutes | Servings: 3

Ingredients:

150G shelled raw king prawns, deveined

2 tsp tamari

2 tsp extra virgin olive oil

75 soba

Directions:

Warm a skillet over high heat, and then fry for the pawns in 1 tsp of the tamari and 1 tsp of olive oil.

Transfer the contents of the skillet to a plate, and then wipe the skillet with a kitchen towel to remove the lingering sauce.

Boil water and cook the soba for 8 minutes, or according to packet directions.

Drain and set aside for later.

Using the remaining 1 tsp olive oil, fry the remaining ingredients for 3-4 minutes.

Add the stock and bring to the boil, simmering until the vegetables are tender but still have bite.

Add the lovage, noodles and prawn intothe skillet, stir, bring back to the boil and then serve.

Miso caramelized tofu

Preparation time: 5 minutes | Cooking time: 40 minutes | Servings: 3

Ingredients:

1 tbsp mirin

20g miso paste

1 x 150g firm tofu

40g celery, trimmed

35g red onion

120g courgette

1 bird's eye chilli

1 garlic clove, finely chopped

1 tsp finely chopped fresh ginger

50g kale, chopped

2 tsp sesame seeds

35g buckwheat

1 tsp ground turmeric

2 tsp extra virgin olive oil

1 tsp tamari (or soy sauce)

Directions:

Preheat your over to 200C or gas mark 6.

Cover a tray with baking parchment.

Combine the mirin and miso together.

Dice the tofu and coat it in the mirin-miso mixture in a resealable plastic bag.

Set aside to marinate.

Chop the vegetables (except for the kale) at a diagonal angle to produce long slices.

Using a steamer, cook for the kale for 5 minutes and set aside.

Disperse the tofu across the lined tray and garnish with sesame seeds.

Roast for 20 minutes, or until caramelized.

Rinse the buckwheat using running water and a sieve.

Add to a pan of boiling water alongside turmeric and cook the buckwheat according to the packet directions.

Heat the oil in a skillet over high heat.

Toss in the vegetables, herbs and spices then fry for 2-3 minutes.

Reduce to medium heat and fry for a further 5 minutes or until cooked but still crunchy.

Sirtfood cauliflower couscous & turkey steak

Preparation time: 5 minutes | Cooking time: 45 minutes | Servings: 3

Ingredients:

150G cauliflower, roughly chopped

1 garlic clove, finely chopped

40g red onion, finely chopped

1 bird's eye chilli, finely chopped

1 tsp finely chopped fresh ginger

2 tbsp extra virgin olive oil

2 tsp ground turmeric

30g sun-dried tomatoes, finely chopped

10g parsley

150G turkey steak

1 tsp dried sage

Juice of ½ lemon

1 tbsp capers

Directions:

Disintegrate the cauliflower using a food processor.

Blend in 1-2 pulses until the cauliflower has a breadcrumb-like consistency.

In a skillet, fry garlic, chilli, ginger and red onion in 1 tsp olive oil for 2-3 minutes.

Throw in the turmeric and cauliflower then cook for another 1-2 minutes.

Remove from heat and add the tomatoes and roughly half the parsley.

Garnish the turkey steak with sage and dress with oil.

In a skillet, over medium heat, fry the turkey steak for 5 minutes, turning occasionally.

Once the steak is cooked, add lemon juice, capers and a dash of water.

Stir and serve with the couscous.

Red onion dhal

Preparation time: 5 minutes | Cooking time: 40 minutes | Servings: 3

Ingredients:

1 tsp extra virgin olive oil

1 tsp mustard seeds

40g red onion, finely chopped

1 garlic clove, finely chopped

1 tsp finely chopped fresh ginger

1 bird's eye chilli, finely chopped

1 tsp mild curry powder

2 tsp ground turmeric

300ml vegetable stock

40g red lentils, rinsed 50g kale

50ml tinned coconut milk

50g buckwheat

Directions:

In a moderately sized saucepan, warm the olive oil over medium heat.

Toss in the mustard seeds and fry until they start to crackle.

Add the garlic, ginger, chilli and onion frying for 10 minutes, or until the onion is tender.

Throw in 1 tsp turmeric and curry powder, and then stir.

Cook for a few minutes until fragrant, then pour in the stock and bring to the boil.

Pour in the lentils and cook for 30 minutes.

Add the coconut milk and kale, cooking for another 5 minutes or so.

As the dhal is brewing, rinse the buckwheat with water and cook it according to packet directions.

Drain and serve with the dhal.

Tofu & shiitake mushroom soup

Preparation time: 5 minutes | Cooking time: 30 minutes | Servings: 3

Ingredients:

10g dried wakame

1L vegetable stock

200g shiitake mushrooms, sliced

120g miso paste

1 x 400g firm tofu, diced

2 green onion, trimmed and diagonally chopped

1 bird's eye chilli, finely chopped

Directions:

Soak the wakame in lukewarm water for 10-15 minutes before draining.

In a medium-sized saucepan add the vegetable stock and bring to the boil.

Toss in the mushrooms and simmer for 2-3 minutes.

Mix the miso paste with 3-4 tbsp of vegetable stock from the saucepan, until the miso is entirely dissolved.

Pour the miso-stock back into the pan and add the tofu, wakame, green onions and chilli, then serve immediately.

Mushroom & tofu scrambled

Preparation time: 5 minutes | Cooking time: 40 minutes | Servings: 3

Ingredients:

100g tofu, extra firm

1 tsp ground turmeric

1 tsp mild curry powder

20g kale, roughly chopped

1 tsp extra virgin olive oil

20g red onion, thinly sliced

50g mushrooms, thinly sliced

5g parsley, finely chopped

Directions:

Place 2 sheets of kitchen towel under and on top of the tofu, then rest a considerable weight such as saucepan onto the tofu, to ensure it drains off the liquid.

Combine the curry powder, turmeric and 1-2 tsp of water to form a paste.

Using a steamer cook kale for 3-4 minutes.

In a skillet, warm oil over medium heat.

Add the chilli, mushrooms and onion, cooking for several minutes or until brown and tender.

Break the tofu into small pieces and toss in the skillet.

Coat with the spice paste and stir, ensuring everything becomes evenly coated.

Cook for up to 5 minutes, or until the tofu has browned then add the kale and fry for 2 more minutes.

Garnish with parsley before serving.

Prawn & chilli pak choi

Preparation time: 5 minutes | Cooking time: 45 minutes | Servings: 3

Ingredients:

75g brown rice

1 pak choi

60ml chicken stock

1 tbsp extra virgin olive oil

1 garlic clove, finely chopped

50g red onion, finely chopped

½ bird's eye chilli, finely chopped

1 tsp freshly grated ginger

125g shelled raw king prawns

1 tbsp soy sauce

1 tsp five-spice

1 tbsp freshly chopped flat-leaf parsley

A pinch of salt and pepper

Directions:

Bring a medium-sized saucepan of water to the boil and cook the brown rice for 25-30 minutes, or until softened.

Tear the pak choi into pieces.

Warm the chicken stock in a skillet over medium heat and toss in the pak choi, cooking until the pak choi has slightly wilted.

In another skillet, warm olive oil over high heat.

Toss in the ginger, chilli, red onions and garlic frying for 2-3 minutes.

Throw in the pawns, five-spice and soy sauce and cook for 6-8 minutes, or until the cooked throughout.

Drain the brown rice and add to the skillet, stirring and cooking for 2-3 minutes.

Add the pak choi, garnish with parsley and serve.

Sirtfood granola

Preparation time: 5 minutes | Cooking time: 30 minutes | Servings: 3

Ingredients:

200g oats

250G buckwheat flakes

100g walnuts, chopped

100g almonds, chopped

100g dried strawberries

1½ tsp ground ginger

1½ tsp ground cinnamon

120ml olive oil

2 tbsp honey

Directions:

Preheat oven to 150C or gas mark 3.

Line a tray with baking parchment.

Stir together walnuts, almonds, buckwheat flakes and oats with ginger and cinnamon.

In a large pan, warm olive oil and honey, heating until the honey has dissolved.

Pour the honey-oil over the other ingredients, stirring to ensuring an even coating.

Separate the granola evenly over the lined baking tray and roast for 50 minutes, or until golden.

Remove from the oven and leave to cool.

Once cooled, add the berries and store in an airtight container.

Eat dry or with milk and yoghurt.

It stays fresh for up to 1 WEEk.

Tomato frittata

Preparation time: 5 minutes | Cooking time: 20 minutes | Servings: 3

Ingredients: 50g cheddar cheese, grated

75g kalamata olives pitted and halved

8 cherry tomatoes, halved 4 large eggs

1 tbsp fresh parsley, chopped

1 tbsp fresh basil, chopped

1 tbsp olive oil

Directions:

Whisk eggs together in a large mixing bowl.

Toss in the parsley, basil, olives, tomatoes and cheese, stirring thoroughly.

In a small skillet, heat the olive oil over high heat.

Pour in the frittata mixture and cook for 5-10 minutes, or set.

Remove the skillet from the hob and place under the grill for 5 minutes, or until firm and set.

Divide into portions and serve immediately.

Horseradish flaked salmon fillet & kale

Preparation time: 5 minutes | Cooking time: 30 minutes | Servings: 3

Ingredients:

200g skinless, boneless salmon fillet

50g green beans

75g kale

1 tbsp extra virgin olive oil

½ garlic clove, crushed

50g red onion, chopped

1 tbsp fresh chives, chopped

1 tbsp freshly chopped flat-leaf parsley

1 tbsp low-fat Crème Fraiche

1Tbsp horseradish sauce

Juice of ¼ lemon

A pinch of salt and pepper

Directions:

Preheat the grill.

Sprinkle a salmon fillet with salt and pepper.

Place under the grill for 10-15 minutes.

Flake and set aside.

Using a steamer, cook the kale and green beans for 10 minutes.

In a skillet, warm the oil over high heat. Add garlic and red onion and fry for 2-3 minutes.

Toss in the kale and beans, and then cook for 1-2 minutes more.

Mix the chives, parsley, Crème Fraiche, horseradish, lemon juice and flaked salmon.

Serve the kale and beans topped with the dressed flaked salmon.

Indulgent yoghurt

Preparation time: 5 minutes | Cooking time: 40 minutes | Servings: 3

Ingredients:

125 mixed berries

150G Greek yoghurt

25 walnuts, chopped

10g dark chocolate (at least 85% cocoa solids), grated

Directions:

Toss the mixed berries into a serving bowl.

Cover with yoghurt and top with chocolate and walnuts.

Sirtfood scrambled eggs

Preparation time: 5 minutes | Cooking time: 40 minutes | Servings: 3

Ingredients: 1 tsp extra virgin olive oil

20g red onion, finely chopped

½ bird's eye chilli, finely chopped

3 medium eggs 50ml milk

1 tsp ground turmeric

5g parsley, finely chopped

Directions: In a skillet, heat the oil over high heat. Toss in the red onion and chilli, frying for 2-3 minutes.

In a large bowl, whisk together the milk, parsley, eggs and turmeric.

Pour into the skillet and lower to medium heat. Cook for 3 to 5 minutes, scrambling the mixture as you do with a spoon or spatula. Serve immediately.

Kale & feta salad

Preparation time: 5 minutes | Cooking time: 40 minutes | Servings: 3

Ingredients:

250G kale, finely chopped

50g walnuts, chopped

75g feta cheese, broken

1 apple, peeled, cored & diced

4 Medjool dates, chopped

75g cranberries

½ red onion, chopped

3 tbsp olive oil

3 tbsp water

2 tsp honey

1 tbsp red wine vinegar

A pinch of salt

Directions:

In a bowl, throw together the kale, walnuts, feta cheese, apple and dates, and then stir.

In a food processor add cranberries, red onion, olive oil, water, honey, red wine vinegar and a pinch of salt.

Process until smooth and fluid, adding water if necessary.

Pour the cranberry dressing over the salad and serve.

Tuna salad

Preparation time: 5 minutes | Cooking time: 40 minutes | Servings: 3

Ingredients:

100g red chicory

150G tuna flakes in brine, drained

100g cucumber

25G rocket

6 kalamata olives, pitted

2 hard-boiled eggs, peeled and quartered

2 tomatoes, chopped

2 tbsp fresh parsley, chopped

1 red onion, chopped

1 celery stalk

1 tbsp capers

2 tbsp garlic vinaigrette

Directions:

Combine all ingredients in a bowl and serve.

Chilli tomato king prawns

Preparation time: 5 minutes | Cooking time: 30 minutes | Servings: 3

Ingredients:

100g (3½oz) pak choi (bok choy)

24 raw king prawns (jumbo shrimp), shelled

4 tomatoes, chopped

2 bird's eye chillies, chopped

1 tbsp fresh coriander (cilantro),chopped

1 tbsp fresh parsley, chopped

2 tbsp olive oil

Directions:

Heat a tbsp of oil in a frying pan and add in the prawns (shrimps) and cook until they are completely pink.

Remove and set aside.

Heat another tbsp of oil in a pan and add the pak choi (bok choy), tomatoes and chilli peppers.

Cook for 3 minutes.

Return the prawns to the pan and warm through.

Sprinkle with chopped parsley and coriander (cilantro) and stir.

Serve with brown rice and salad.

Air-fried French toast sticks

Preparation time: 5 minutes | Cooking time: 40 minutes | Servings: 3

Ingredients:

4 eggs

½ cup milk

¼ tsp vanilla concentrate

¼ tsp ground cinnamon

1/3 cup granulated sugar

6 cuts white bread, cut in thirds

Maple syrup

Directions:

In a little bowl, whisk together eggs, milk, vanilla concentrate, cinnamon, and sugar. Coat air fry bin generously with cooking splash.

Working each, in turn, plunge each bit of bread in the egg blend, at that point move to the bushel.

Select air fry set the temperature to 400F and set time to 10 minutes.

Press start/pause to start preheating.

At the point when the unit has preheated, slide container into the upper rails of the stove.

Following 5 minutes, press start/pause to delay the unit.

Expel crate from the stove.

Utilizing tongs, flip each bit of bread.

At that point, pivot container 180F.

Return container to the broiler, and press start/pause to continue cooking for 5 additional minutes.

When cooking is finished, expel bin from broiler.

Sprinkle maple syrup over French toast sticks and serve.

Toasted ravioli

Preparation time: 5 minutes | Cooking time: 25 minutes | Servings: 3

Ingredients:

20 solidified ravioli

1 cup universally handy flour

3 eggs, whisked

¼ cup olive oil

2 cups Italian-style panko breadcrumbs

1 cup marinara sauce

Directions:

Spot flour in a blending bowl.

Spot eggs in another bowl.

In a third bowl, consolidate olive oil with panko breadcrumbs and blend all together.

Working in groups, hurl ravioli in flour.

Shake off overabundance flour, at that point dunk ravioli in eggs.

Move ravioli to breadcrumbs and coat well.

Put in a safe spot.

Spot the cook and crisp basket in the pot.

Close crisping cover. Preheat the unit by choosing air crisp, setting the temperature to 375F, and setting the opportunity to 5 minutes.

Following 5 minutes, open the crisping cover and spot a large portion of the ravioli in the bushel.

Close top. Select air crisp, set the temperature to 375F and set time to 10 minutes.

Select start/stop to start.

When cooking is finished, move ravioli to a serving dish.

Spot remaining ravioli in the bin and rehash stages 5 and 6.

When cooking is finished, serve ravioli with marinara sauce.

Pierogi

Preparation time: 5 minutes | Cooking time: 30 minutes | Servings: 3

Ingredients:

2 cups of water

2 pounds solidified pierogi (approx. 2 boxes)

2 tbsp olive oil

¼ cup acrid cream

1 tbsp crisp chives, hacked (discretionary)

Directions:

Empty water into the pot, at that point, embed the cook and crisp basket.

Spot the pierogi in the bin.

Gather pressure top, ensuring the weight discharge valve is in the vent position.

Select steam and set time to 10 minutes.

Select start/stop to start.

When steaming is finished, move pierogi to a blending bowl and hurl it with olive oil.

At that point move pierogi back to the bin.

Close the crisping cover.

Select air crisp, set the temperature to 375F and set time to 20 minutes.

Press start/stop to start.

Following 10 minutes, open cover, at that point lift container and shake pierogi.

Lower container once again into the pot and close top to continue cooking.

When cooking is finished, move pierogi to a serving dish and present with acrid cream bested with chives, whenever wanted.

Pasta salad

Preparation time: 5 minutes | Cooking time: 40 minutes | Servings: 3

Ingredients:

A plate of mixed greens ingredients

1 box (16 ounces) elbow pasta

4 cups of water

1 tbsp fit salt

2 tbsp olive oil

½ cup red onion, diced

1 cup simmered red peppers, daintily cut

¼ cup dark olives, cut

½ pound (8 ounces) crisp mozzarella, diced

½ cup slashed basil

Red wine vinaigrette ingredients

1 box (16 ounces) elbow pasta

4 cups of water

1 tbsp fit salt

2 tbsp olive oil

½ cup red onion, diced

1 cup simmered red peppers, daintily cut

¼ cup dark olives, cut

½ pound (8 ounces) crisp mozzarella, diced

½ cup slashed basil

Directions:

Amass pressure top, ensuring the weight discharge valve is in the seal position.

Select pressure and set it to high. Set time to 3 minutes.

Select start/stop to start.

While the pasta is cooking, set up the red wine vinaigrette.

In a blending bowl, join all vinaigrette fixings aside from olive oil.

Gradually speed in the olive oil until completely joined.

Taste and alter seasonings as wanted.

Put in a safe spot.

At the point when weight cooking is finished, enable the strain to normally discharge for 10 minutes.

Following 10 minutes, snappy discharge remaining weight by moving the weight discharge valve to the vent position.

Cautiously expel top when the unit has completed the process of discharging pressure.

Evacuate the pot and strain the pasta in a colander.

Move to a bowl and hurl with 2 tbsp of olive oil.

Spot bowl in cooler and enable pasta to cool for 20 minutes.

When pasta has cooled, mix in red onion, broiled peppers, dark olives, mozzarella, and basil.

Delicately crease in the red wine vinaigrette.

Serve quickly, or cover and refrigerate for serving later.

Meat tacos with hidden veggies

Preparation time: 5 minutes | Cooking time: 20 minutes | Servings: 3

Ingredients:

2 tbsp olive oil, partitioned

1 red chile pepper, cut

1 green chile pepper, cut

1 yellow onion, stripped, cut

1 bundle (16 ounces) shaved steak

2 tbsp garlic powder

1 tbsp ground cumin

2 tbsp genuine salt

1 tsp ground dark pepper

1 bundle corn tortilla

1 sack (16 ounces) destroyed cheddar

Directions:

Following 5 minutes, include 1 tbsp olive oil and ringer peppers to the pot.

Sauté peppers, mixing at times, until cooked through, around 5 minutes.

Expel peppers from pot and put them in a safe spot.

To collect tacos, place a limited quantity of cooked peppers in every tortilla.

Spread the peppers with steak.

At that point top with cheddar and any of your other most loved garnishes and serve.

Beef with quinoa and melting onions

Preparation time: 5 minutes | Cooking time: 20 minutes | Servings: 3

Ingredients:

2Lb stewing beef (grass-fed)

1 cup quinoa, rinsed

4 large onions, sliced

3 garlic cloves, chopped

1 bay leaf

2 cups chicken broth

4 tbsp extra virgin olive oil

1 tsp cinnamon

½ tsp ginger powder

Salt and black pepper, to taste

Directions:

Heat olive oil in a large saucepan and brown the beef.

Add in the onions and garlic and saute for 2-3 minutes, stirring.

Add in cinnamon, ginger, the bay leaf, black pepper and chicken broth.

Bring to a boil.

Reduce heat to low, cover, and simmer for about 90 minutes, stirring occasionally.

When the beef is almost done, add in quinoa, stir and simmer for 20 minutes more.

Skillet chickpeas with broccoli

Preparation time: 5 minutes | Cooking time: 40 minutes | Servings: 3

Ingredients:

1 can chickpeas

12 oz broccoli florets

3 garlic cloves, chopped

1 can tomatoes (15 oz), diced anddrained

1Lb bag baby spinach

2 tbsp extra virgin olive oil

4 eggs

salt and pepper, to taste

Directions:

Heat olive oil in a cast-iron skillet over medium-high heat.

Gently sauté garlic for 1 minute, or until just fragrant.

Add chickpeas, tomatoes and broccoli and stir to combine.

Cook for about ten minutes or until broccoli is tender.

Add spinach, and stir to combine.

Break the eggs over chickpea mixture.

Place skillet in the oven and bake at 350F for 15 minutes.

Kale, edamame and tofu curry

Preparation time: 5 minutes | Cooking time: 40 minutes | Servings: 3

Ingredients:

1 tbsp rapeseed oil

1 huge onion, slashed

4 cloves garlic, stripped and ground

1 huge thumb (7cm) crisp ginger, stripped and ground

1 red stew, deseeded and meagerly cut

½ tsp ground turmeric

¼ tsp cayenne pepper

1 tsp paprika

½ tsp ground cumin

1 tsp salt

250G dried red lentils

1L bubbling water

50g solidified soya-edamame beans

200g firm tofu, hacked into shapes

2 tomatoes, generally hacked

Juice of 1 lime

200g kale leaves stalks expelled and torn

Directions:

Put the oil in an overwhelming bottomed skillet over a low-medium warmth.

Include the onion and cook for 5 minutes before including the garlic, ginger and bean stew and cooking for a further 2 minutes.

Include the turmeric, cayenne, paprika, cumin and salt.

Mix through before including the red lentils and blending once more.

Pour in the bubbling water and bring to a healthy stew for 10 minutes, then lessen the warmth and cook for a further 20-30 minutes until the curry has a thick porridge consistency.

Add the soya beans, tofu and tomatoes and cook for a further 5 minutes.

Include the lime juice and kale leaves and cook until the kale is simply delicate.

Sweet-smelling chicken breast with kale, red onion, and salsa

Preparation time: 5 minutes | Cooking time: 60 minutes | Servings: 3

Ingredients:

120g skinless, boneless chicken bosom

2 tsp ground turmeric

Juice of ¼ lemon

1 tbsp additional virgin olive oil

50g kale slashed

20g red onion, cut

1 tsp slashed new ginger

50g buckwheat

Directions:

To make the salsa, expel the eye from the tomato and slash it finely, taking consideration to keep however much of the fluid as could reasonably be expected.

Blend in with the bean stew, tricks, parsley and lemon juice.

You could place everything in a blender, yet the final product is somewhat different.

Warmth the broiler to 220C/gas 7.

Marinate the chicken bosom in 1 tsp of the turmeric, the lemon juice and a little oil. Leave for 5–10 minutes.

Warmth an ovenproof griddle until hot, then include the marinated chicken and cook for a moment or so on each side, until pale brilliant, then exchange to the broiler (place on a preparing plate if your skillet isn't ovenproof) for 8–10 minutes or until cooked through.

Expel from the broiler, spread with foil and leave to rest for 5 minutes before serving.

In the meantime, cook the kale in a steamer for 5 minutes.

Fry the red onions and the ginger in a little oil, until delicate however not shaded, then include the cooked kale and fry for one more moment.

Cook the buckwheat according to the parcel directions with the rest of the tsp of turmeric.

Serve nearby the chicken, vegetables and salsa.

Salmon sirt super salad

Preparation time: 5 minutes | Cooking time: 40 minutes | Servings: 3

Ingredients:

50g rocket

50g chicory leaves

100g smoked salmon cuts (you can likewise utilize lentils, cooked chicken bosom or tinned fish)

80g avocado, stripped, stoned and cut

40g celery, cut

20g red onion, cut

15G pecans, hacked

1 tbs tricks

1 huge Medjool date, hollowed and slashed

1 tbs extra-virgin olive oil

Juice ¼ lemon

10g parsley, cleaved

10g lovage or celery leaves, cleaved

Directions:

Organize the serving of mixed greens leaves on a huge plate.

Combine all the rest of the fixings and serve over the leaves.

Potato salad recipe

Preparation time: 5 minutes | Cooking time: 35 minutes | Servings: 3

Ingredients:

6 tbsp mayonnaise (or plain yoghurt)

1 tbsp lemon juice

½ tsp salt

Touch of naturally ground dark pepper

2 sweet apples, cored and hacked

1 cup red seedless grapes, cut down the middle (or ¼ cup of raisins)

1 cup celery, meagerly cut

1 cup cleaved, marginally toasted pecans

Lettuce

Roasted eggplant wedges with walnut and parsley pesto and tomato salad

Creamy avocado and chicken spaghetti

Preparation time: 5 minutes | Cooking time: 40 minutes | Servings: 3

Ingredients:

12 oz spaghetti

1 cup cooked chicken, shredded

2 avocados, peeled and diced

1 cup cherry tomatoes, halved

1 garlic clove, chopped

2 tbsp basil pesto

5 tbsp olive oil

4 tbsp lemon juice

¼ cup grated parmesan cheese

Directions:

In a large pot of boiling salted water, cook spaghetti according to package directions. Drain and set aside in a large bowl.

In a blender, combine lemon juice, garlic, basil pesto and avocados and blend until smooth.

Combine spaghetti, chicken, cherry tomatoes and avocado sauce.

Sprinkle with parmesan cheese and serve immediately.

Creamy cauliflower spaghetti

Preparation time: 5 minutes | Cooking time: 45 minutes | Servings: 3

Ingredients:

12 oz spaghetti

3 cups chopped cauliflower

3 cans (28 oz) crushed tomatoes

3 garlic cloves, chopped

1 tsp dried basil

3 tbsp olive oil

¼ cup grated parmesan cheese

Directions:

In a large pot of boiling salted water, cook spaghetti according to package directions. Drain and set aside in a large bowl.

Heat the olive oil over medium heat in a large saucepan and sauté the garlic, onion, and cauliflower, stirring, until the cauliflower is browned and tender, about 35-40 minutes. Add in basil, black pepper, and tomatoes, and simmer until the sauce is thickened and the flavours haveblended.

Combine spaghetti and cauliflower sauce.

Sprinkle with parmesan cheese and serve immediately.

Avocado, roasted mushroom and ham spaghetti

Preparation time: 5 minutes | Cooking time: 40 minutes | Servings: 3

Ingredients:

12 oz spaghetti

1 cup ham, cut in cubes

2 avocados, peeled and diced

10-15 white mushrooms, halved

2 tbsp green olive paste

2 garlic cloves, chopped

Olive oil spray

Salt and black pepper, to taste

¼ cup grated parmesan cheese

Directions:

Line a baking tray with baking paper and place mushrooms on it.

Spray with olive oil and season with salt and black pepper to taste.

Roast in a preheated to 375F oven for 15 minutes, or until golden and tender.

In a large pot of boiling salted water, cook spaghetti according to package directions. Drain and set aside in a large bowl.

In a blender, combine lemon juice, garlic, olive paste and avocados and blend until smooth.

Combine pasta, diced ham, mushrooms and avocado sauce.

Sprinkle with parmesan cheese and serve immediately.

Baked pasta with ham, broccoli and cheese

Preparation time: 5 minutes | Cooking time: 40 minutes | Servings: 3

Ingredients:

2 cups small pasta

1 cup diced ham

1 onion, finely chopped

4 garlic cloves, chopped

3 white button mushrooms, chopped

1 head broccoli, cut in florets

salt and black pepper, to taste

1 cup mozzarella cheese, grated

1 egg, whisked

Directions:

Prepare pasta according to package directions.

Drain and place in an ovenproof casserole.

Heat olive oil in a large skillet and sauté onion until transparent.

Add in mushrooms, garlic and broccoli, stir, and cook on medium heat for about 10 minutes, stirring.

Combine broccoli and mushroom mixture with pasta and ham.

Season with salt and pepper to taste.

Whisk the egg with mozzarella cheese and spread all over the pasta equally.

Bake in a preheated to 350F oven for 15 minutes, or until the cheese turns golden.

Cauliflower casserole

Preparation time: 5 minutes | Cooking time: 40 minutes | Servings: 3

Ingredients:

1 head cauliflower, cut in small florets

1 large red pepper, chopped

1 onion, finely chopped

4 garlic cloves, chopped

1 tsp dried thyme

2 tbsp extra virgin olive oil

8 oz shredded cheddar cheese, divided

8 oz shredded Monterey jack cheese, divided

1 cup sour cream

salt and black pepper, to taste

Directions:

Steam cauliflower florets until tender, about 8 minutes.

Heat olive oil in a large skillet and sauté onion, garlic and the red pepper until fragrant. Stir in thyme.

Stir cauliflower and onion mixture together in an ovenproof casserole.

Season with salt and pepper to taste.

Combine sour cream, 6 oz of the shredded cheddar and 6 oz of the Monterey jack and stir it in the casserole.

Sprinkle on top remaining cheddar and Monterey jack cheese.

Cover the casserole with foil and bake for 25 minutes, remove foil and bake until cheese is brown and bubbly.

Chicken and cauliflower casserole

Preparation time: 5 minutes | Cooking time: 40 minutes | Servings: 3

Ingredients:

½ head cauliflower, cut in small florets

2 cups cooked chicken, diced

6-7 spring onions, finely cut

10-12 cherry tomatoes, halved

½ tsp dried oregano

1Lb oz shredded cheddar cheese, divided

1 cup sour cream

2 tbsp extra virgin olive oil

salt and black pepper, to taste

Directions:

Steam cauliflower florets until tender, about 8 minutes.

Heat olive oil in a large skillet and sauté onions for 1-2 minutes.

Stir in chicken and oregano and cook for 1 minute, stirring.

Combine cauliflower and chicken mixture together in an ovenproof casserole.

Add cherry tomatoes and season with salt and pepper to taste.

Combine sour cream and 6 oz of the shredded cheddar and stir it in the casserole. Sprinkle on top remaining cheddar.

Cover the casserole with foil and bake for 25 minutes, remove foil and bake until cheese is brown and bubbly.

Delicious mushroom tofu pizza

Preparation time: 5 minutes | Cooking time: 50 minutes | Servings: 3

Ingredients:

1 store-bought or homemade dough

2-3 green onions, chopped

10 white button mushrooms, chopped

1 red bell pepper, chopped

½ cup tomato sauce

1 cup of tofu pieces

2 tbsp extra virgin olive oil

½ tsp dried oregano

1 tsp dried thyme

½ tsp garlic powder

salt and black pepper, to taste

2-3 cups mozzarella cheese, shredded

Directions:

In a large skillet, heat olive oil and gently sauté green onions and bell pepper for 4-5 minutes until slightly charred.

Add in the tofu pieces, mushrooms, garlic powder, oregano and thyme and sauté for 5 minutes more.

Season with salt and black pepper to taste.

Roll out dough onto a floured surface and transfer to a round baking sheet lined with parchment paper or an oiled pizza stone.

Top with tomato sauce and the sautéed tofu and mushroom mixture.

Sprinkle with shredded mozzarella cheese.

Bake for about 15 minutes, until the crust is golden brown and the cheese is completely melted.

Let rest for 3-4 minutes before cutting, then serve immediately.

Cauliflower with chilli and mustard

Preparation time: 5 minutes | Cooking time: 40 minutes | Servings: 3

Ingredients:

2Lbs cauliflower, cut into small florets

3 long fresh green chillies, thinly sliced

1 onion, finely chopped

2 garlic cloves, crushed

½ cup vegetable broth

2 tsp mustard seeds

1 tsp ground turmeric

1 tsp tamarind paste

2 tbsp extra virgin olive oil

Directions:

Heat the oil in a large saucepan over medium heat.

Add in the onion and gently saute, stirring, for 3-4 minutes until transparent.

Add in garlic and chilli, and cook for 1 minute until just fragrant.

Add the mustard seeds and turmeric and saute, stirring, for 20 seconds or until the mustard seeds pop.

Add the cauliflower and stir to coat.

Add the vegetable broth and tamarind paste and simmer for 4 minutes or until the cauliflower is tender-crisp.

Season with salt to taste and serve.

Balsamic roasted carrots and baby onions

Preparation time: 5 minutes | Cooking time: 30 minutes | Servings: 3

Ingredients:

2 bunches baby carrots, scrubbed, ends trimmed

10 small onions, peeled, halved

4 tbsp brown sugar

1 tsp thyme

2 tbsp extra virgin olive oil

Directions:

Preheat oven to 350F.

Line a baking tray with baking paper.

Place the carrots, onions, thyme and oil in a large bowl and toss until well coated. Arrange carrots and onions, in a single layer, on the baking tray.

Roast for 20 minutes or until tender.

Sprinkle over the sugar and vinegar and toss to coat.

Roast for 20 minutes more or until the vegetables are tender and caramelized.

Season with salt and pepper to taste and serve.

Roasted artichoke hearts

Preparation time: 5 minutes | Cooking time: 40 minutes | Servings: 3

Ingredients:

2 cans artichoke hearts

4 garlic cloves, quartered

2 tsp extra virgin olive oil

1 tsp dried oregano

salt and pepper, to taste

2-3 tbsp lemon juice, to serve

Directions:

Preheat oven to 375F.

Drain the artichoke hearts and rinse them very well.

Toss them in garlic, oregano and olive oil.

Arrange the artichoke hearts in a baking dish and bake for about 45 minutes tossing a few times if desired.

Season with salt and pepper and serve with lemon juice.

Vegetable quinoa stew

Preparation time: 5 minutes | Cooking time: 20 minutes | Servings: 3

Ingredients:

1 cup quinoa

1½ cup of water

1 onion, finely cut

2 red bell peppers, chopped

1 zucchini, peeled and chopped

1 cup fresh green peas

5-6 green beans

1 tomato, chopped

1 potato, peeled and diced

2 garlic cloves, chopped

1 tbsp paprika

3 tbsp extra virgin olive oil

salt, to taste

½ cup fresh dill, finely cut, to serve

Directions:

Rinse the quinoa very well in a sieve under running water and set aside to drain.

Heat olive oil in a large saucepan over medium-high heat.

Add in the onion and sauté for 1-2 minutes.

Add the garlic, paprika, bell pepper, green peas, green beans and zucchini.

Cook, occasionally stirring, for 5 minutes then add the tomato, the potato, and the water.

Bring to the boil and add in quinoa.

Stir, cover, and cook for 20 minutes.

Season with salt to taste and serve sprinkled with dill.

Ground beef, quinoa and cabbage casserole

Preparation time: 5 minutes | Cooking time: 60 minutes | Servings: 3

Ingredients:

1Lb ground beef

1 cup quinoa, rinsed

½ cabbage, shredded

½ onion, chopped

2 leeks, white part only, chopped

1 tomato, diced

1 tbsp paprika

½ tsp cumin

½ tsp black pepper

4 tbsp extra virgin olive oil

salt, to taste

Directions:

In a deep saucepan, sauté the onion and leeks in olive oil until tender.

Add in the ground beef, quinoa, tomato, paprika, cumin, salt and black pepper.

Stir very well.

Place shredded cabbage on the bottom of an ovenproof baking dish.

Cover with beef and quinoa mixture.

Cover with a lid or aluminium foil and bake at 325F for 40 minutes.

Citrus pork with quinoa

Preparation time: 5 minutes | Cooking time: 40 minutes | Servings: 3

Ingredients:

1Lb pork shoulder, cut into 1-inch chunks

1 cup quinoa, rinsed

1 cup of orange juice

1 cup of water

1 large carrot, chopped

6-7 spring onions, finely cut

1-2 garlic cloves, chopped

1 tbsp lemon zest

½ tsp cumin

3 tbsp extra virgin olive oil

Directions:

Heat the olive oil in a large skillet over medium-high heat.

Working in batches, brown the pieces of pork shoulder.

Add in the carrots, garlic, lemon zest, cumin, salt and black pepper to taste.

Stir, and cook for 1-2 minutes, stirring.

Add the orange juice and water, bring to a simmer and cook for 40 minutes.

Stir in quinoa and spring onions and cook for 15 minutes more.

Comforting lamb and quinoa shepherd's stew

Preparation time: 5 minutes | Cooking time: 45 minutes | Servings: 3

Ingredients:

4 shoulder lamb chops, de-boned and cubed

1 cup quinoa

1½ cups chicken broth

1 onion, finely cut

2 garlic cloves, chopped

2 red peppers, chopped

1 carrot, cut into bite-size pieces

1 turnip, cut into bite-size pieces

6-7 white mushrooms, chopped

1-2 tomatoes, diced

2 tbsp extra virgin olive oil

1 tbsp paprika

1 bay leaf

1 tbsp thyme

Directions:

Wash quinoa very well, drain and set aside.

In a large soup pot or casserole dish, heat the oil over medium heat and brown the meat for 8-10 minutes.

Add the onion, bell peppers and garlic and cook until softened, about 3 minutes.

Stir in paprika, the bay leaf and thyme.

Add the other vegetables and mushrooms and cook for 1-2 minutes, stirring.

Add in the broth, bring to the boil and simmer for 30 minutes.

Stir in the quinoa and simmer for 15 minutes more.

Tuna and quinoa patties

Preparation time: 5 minutes | Cooking time: 30 minutes | Servings: 3

Ingredients:

2 6 oz cans tuna

½ cup cooked quinoa

1 large egg

1 tbsp dijon mustard

2 tbsp lemon juice

2-3 spring onions, finely chopped

½ cup fresh parsley, finely chopped

¼ cup extra virgin olive oil

1 tsp salt

Black pepper, to taste

Directions:

In a medium bowl, mix together the tuna, mustard, quinoa, lemon juice, spring onions, parsley, and salt.

Add in freshly ground black pepper andthe egg.

Using your hands, form batter into burgers.

Bake in a preheated to 375F oven for 7-8 minutes or until golden.

Spicy chickpea and spinach stew

Preparation time: 5 minutes | Cooking time: 50 minutes | Servings: 3

Ingredients:

1 onion, chopped

3 garlic cloves, chopped

1 15 oz can chickpeas, drained and rinsed

1 15 oz can of tomatoes, diced and undrained

1 1LB bag baby spinach

A handful of blanched almonds

½ cup vegetable broth

1 tbsp hot chilli paste

½ tsp cumin

salt and pepper, to taste

Directions:

Heat olive oil in a large saucepan over medium-high heat.

Gently sauté onion and garlic for 4-5 minutes, or until tender.

Add spices and stir.

Add in chickpeas, tomatoes, almonds and broth.

Bring to a boil, then reduce heat to low and simmer, partially covered, for 10 minutes.

Add the chilli paste and spinach to the pot and stir until the spinach wilts.

Remove from heat and season with salt and pepper to taste.

Moroccan chickpea stew

Preparation time: 5 minutes | Cooking time: 20 minutes | Servings: 3

Ingredients: 1 onion, chopped

3 garlic cloves, chopped

2 large carrots, chopped

2 sweet potatoes, peeled and chopped

4-5 dates, pitted and chopped

1 cup spinach, chopped

1 15 oz can of tomatoes, diced and undrained

1 15 oz can chickpeas, rinsed and drained

1 cup vegetable broth

1 tbsp ground cumin

½ tsp chilli powder

½ tsp ground turmeric

½ tsp salt

3 tbsp extra virgin olive oil

½ cup chopped cilantro, to serve

grated lemon zest, to serve

Directions:

Heat olive oil in a large saucepan over medium-high heat.

Gently sauté onion, garlic and carrots for 4-5 minutes, or until tender.

Add all spices and stir.

Stir in all other ingredients except the spinach.

Bring to a boil, cover, reduce heat, and simmer for 20 minutes, or until potatoes are tender.

Add in spinach, stir and cook it until it wilts.

Serve over brown rice, quinoa or couscous and top with chopped cilantro and lemon zest.

Baked falafels

Preparation time: 5 minutes | Cooking time: 20 minutes | Servings: 3

Ingredients:

1 can chickpeas, drained and rinsed

1 small carrot, cut

1 onion, cut

2 garlic cloves, minced

½ cup fresh parsley, finely cut

¼ cup whole wheat flour

¼ cup tahini

¼ cup extra virgin olive oil

2-3 tbsp lemon juice

2 tsp cumin (or to taste)

1 tsp salt

Black pepper, to taste

Directions:

Blend the carrots, chickpeas, onion and garlic in a food processor until completely minced. When it turns to a smooth paste, add in parsley and transfer to a large mixing bowl.

Stir in the remaining ingredients.

Using a large tbsp form batter into burgers.

Bake in a preheated to 375F oven until golden.

Conclusion

According to nutritionists Aidan Goggins and Glen Matten, who have developed the sirtfood diet, the consumption of certain foods would activate sirtuins, a group of genes that stimulate the metabolism, burn fat and promote rapid weight loss.

According to the studies developed by the two doctors, these genes stimulate the metabolism, cause fat burning and promote a fairly rapid weight loss. In addition, sirtuins are able to repair cells and improve general health by transforming from slimming instruments to elixirs of longevity.

I hope this guide has helped you become acquainted with the sirtfood diet and achieve your weight loss and health goals. Good luck on your sirtfood journey!

CPSIA information can be obtained
at www.ICGtesting.com
Printed in the USA
LVHW020026100221
678894LV00013B/939